DATE DUE

Allografts

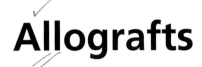

Guest Editor

DARREN L. JOHNSON, MD

CLINICS IN
SPORTS MEDICINE

www.sportsmed.theclinics.com

Consulting Editor
MARK D. MILLER, MD

April 2009 • Volume 28 • Number 2

SAUNDERS an imprint of ELSEVIER, Inc.

W.B. SAUNDERS COMPANY
A Division of Elsevier Inc.

1600 John F. Kennedy Blvd. • Suite 1800 • Philadelphia, Pennsylvania 19103
http://www.theclinics.com

CLINICS IN SPORTS MEDICINE Volume 28, Number 2
April 2009 ISSN 0278-5919, ISBN-13: 978-1-4377-0543-0, ISBN-10: 1-4377-0543-X
Editor: Ruth Malwitz

Clinics in Sports Medicine (ISSN 0278-5919) is published quarterly by Elsevier Inc., 360 Park Avenue South, New York, NY 10010-1710. Months of publication are January, April, July, and October. Business and Editorial Offices: 1600 John F. Kennedy Blvd., Suite 1800, Philadelphia, PA 19103-2899. Customer Service Offices: 6277 Sea Harbor Drive, Orlando, FL 32887-4800. Periodicals postage paid at New York, NY, and additional mailing offices. Subscription prices are $253.00 per year (US individuals), $393.00 per year (US institutions), $127.00 per year (US students), $286.00 per year (Canadian individuals), $475.00 per year (Canadian institutions), $177.00 (Canadian students), $347.00 per year (foreign individuals), $475.00 per year (foreign institutions), and $177.00 per year (foreign students). Foreign air speed delivery is included in all *Clinics* subscription prices. All prices are subject to change without notice. **POSTMASTER:** Send address changes to *Clinics in Sports Medicine*, Elsevier Periodicals Customer Service, 11830 Westline Industrial Drive, St. Louis, MO 63146. Customer Service (orders, claims, online, change of address): Elsevier Periodicals Customer Service, 11830 Westline Industrial Drive, St. Louis, MO 63146. Tel: 1-800-654-2452 (U.S. and Canada); 314-453-7041 (outside U.S. and Canada). Fax: 314-453-5170. E-mail: journalscustomerservice-usa@elsevier.com (for print support); journalsonlinesupport-usa@elsevier.com (for online support).

Reprints. For copies of 100 or more of articles in this publication, please contact the Commercial Reprints Department, Elsevier Inc., 360 Park Avenue South, New York, NY 10010-1710. Tel.: 212-633-3812; Fax: 212-462-1935; E-mail: reprints@elsevier.com.

Clinics in Sports Medicine is covered in *MEDLINE/PubMed (Index Medicus) Current Contents/Clinical Medicine, Excerpta Medica,* and *ISI/Biomed.*

Printed in the United States of America.

Contributors

CONSULTING EDITOR

MARK D. MILLER, MD
S. Ward Casscells Professor of Orthopaedic Surgery; Head, Division of Sports Medicine, University of Virginia; Team Physician, James Madison University, Charlottesville, Virginia

GUEST EDITOR

DARREN L. JOHNSON, MD
Professor and Chairman, Department of Orthopaedic Surgery; Director of Sports Medicine, Department of Orthopaedic Surgery, University of Kentucky, Lexington, Kentucky

AUTHORS

ANNUNZIATO AMENDOLA, MD
Professor, Department of Orthopaedic Surgery; Director, University of Iowa Sports Medicine, University of Iowa Health Care, Iowa City, Iowa

FREDERICK M. AZAR, MD
Professor; Director, Sports Medicine Fellowship; Director, Residency Program, University of Tennessee-Campbell Clinic Department of Orthopaedic Surgery, Memphis, Tennessee

GENE R. BARRETT, MD
Clinical Professor, Mississippi Sports Medicine and Orthopaedic Center, Jackson, Mississippi

J.C. CLARK, MD
Orthopaedic Surgery Resident, University of Florida Orthopaedic and Sports Medicine Institute, Gainesville, Florida

RYAN D. DELLAMAGGIORA, MD
Department of Orthopaedic Surgery, University of Southern California, Keck School of Medicine, Healthcare Consultation Center, Los Angeles, California

MICHAEL J. EAGAN, MD
Resident Physician, UCLA Department of Orthopaedic Surgery, David Geffen School of Medicine at UCLA, Los Angeles, California

CHRISTOPHER D. HARNER, MD
Blue Cross of Western Pennsylvania Professor; Medical Director, UPMC Sports Performance Complex, UPMC Center for Sports Medicine, Department of Orthopaedic Surgery, University of Pittsburgh Medical Center, Pittsburgh, Pennsylvania

ANDREW D. HEINZELMANN, MD
Fellow, Mississippi Sports Medicine and Orthopaedic Center, Jackson, Mississippi

PETER A. INDELICATO, MD
Wayne Huizenga Professor of Sports Medicine; Division Chief, Sports Medicine; Head
Team Physician, UF Athletic Association, University of Florida, Gainesville, Florida

DARREN L. JOHNSON, MD
Professor and Chairman, Department of Orthopaedic Surgery; Director of Sports
Medicine, Department of Orthopaedic Surgery, University of Kentucky, Lexington,
Kentucky

DAVID M. JUNKIN, Jr., MD
Clinical Sports Medicine Fellow, Department of Orthopaedic Surgery, University
of Kentucky, Orthopaedic Specialty Center, Willow Grove, Pennsylvania

CHRISTIAN LATTERMANN, MD
Assistant Professor and Director of Cartilage Repair and Restoration, University
of Kentucky, Department of Orthopaedic Surgery and Sports Medicine, Lexington,
Kentucky

MARVIN Y. LO, MD
Clinical Fellow, UPMC Sports Performance Complex, UPMC Center for Sports Medicine,
Department of Orthopaedic Surgery, University of Pittsburgh Medical Center, Pittsburgh,
Pennsylvania; Orthopaedic Group of San Francisco, San Francisco, California

DAVID R. McALLISTER, MD
Associate Professor and Chief of Sports Medicine, UCLA Department of Orthopaedic
Surgery, David Geffen School of Medicine at UCLA, Los Angeles, California

MICHAEL MOSER, MD
Assistant Professor, Sports Medicine; Team Physician, UF Athletic Association,
University of Florida, Gainesville, Florida

JONATHAN D. PACKER, MD
Laboratory for Soft Tissue Research, Hospital for Special Surgery, New York,
New York

SCOTT A. RODEO, MD
Co-Chief, Sports Medicine and Shoulder Service; Professor, Orthopaedic Surgery,
Weill Medical College of Cornell University, The Hospital for Special Surgery, New York,
New York

SPENCER E. ROMINE, MD
Resident Physician, University of Kentucky, Department of Orthopaedic Surgery
and Sports Medicine, Lexington, Kentucky

ROBERT N. ROYALTY, MD
Resident Physician, Department of Orthopaedic Surgery, University of Kentucky,
Lexington, Kentucky

DANIEL E. RUEFF, MD
Orthopaedic Surgery Resident, University of Florida Orthopaedic and Sports Medicine
Institute, Gainesville, Florida

WALTER R. SHELTON, MD
Mississippi Sports Medicine and Orthopaedic Center, Jackson, Mississippi

MARY P. STOLLEY, RN BSN
Clinical Research Coordinator, Department of Orthopaedic Surgery, University of Iowa Health Care, Iowa City, Iowa

C. THOMAS VANGSNESS, Jr., MD
Professor of Orthopaedics, Department of Orthopaedic Surgery, University of Southern California, Keck School of Medicine, Healthcare Consultation Center, Los Angeles, California

Contents

Allografts used in orthopedic surgery have steadily increased. With concerns regarding tissue safety and processing, governing entities have increased their regulation. This review articles discusses current testing and processing of allografts as well as the rules of their handling.

Secondary sterilization of musculoskeletal allografts may use chemicals, radiation, or combinations of these. No sterilization techniques have been definitively proven to be more effective than others, and their biomechanical and biological effects on allograft tissue remain largely unknown. The current risk of an allograft infection appears to be much less than the risk of infection surrounding the surgical procedure itself. With appropriate donor screening, improved donor testing—including nucleic acid testing (NAT), and adherence to AATB standards—the risk of disease transmission or infections can be eliminated or substantially decreased.

The use of implantation of allograft tissue in sports medicine has risen steadily over the last decade. Allograft tissues offer several advantages over autografts, including reduced donor-site morbidity and decreased operative time, and in some instances, no autograft option exists. However, with allografts, there is a small risk of disease transmission, immunologic rejection, and decreased biologic incorporation. Several techniques to limit these pitfalls and maximize graft incorporation are available, however. This chapter takes an in-depth look at the biology of allograft incorporation and how these techniques affect graft incorporation.v

The use of allografts in sports medicine is becoming increasingly popular, and, therefore, this issue of *Clinics in Sports Medicine* is dedicated to the use of allografts in sports medicine. The majority of indications are related to the use of soft tissue grafts for ligament reconstruction, osteochondral (OC) allografts for articular surface reconstruction, and meniscal allografts for meniscal transplantation. There is an increasing amount of science and literature dealing with healing and outcomes, but many questions still remain. There are a number of issues, controversies, and lack of long-term outcomes to make definitive statements on what is really known about allograft use in sports medicine.

While bone-patellar tendon-bone (BPTB) autograft continues to be the "gold standard" and most popular graft choice for primary anterior cruciate ligament (ACL) reconstructions, the use of allograft tissues in ACL reconstruction has steadily increased over the last 2 decades. Advantages of allograft include a lack of donor-site morbidity, unlimited available sizes, shorter operative times, availability of larger grafts, smaller incisions, improved cosmesis, lower incidence of postoperative arthrofibrosis, faster immediate postoperative recovery, and less postoperative pain. Disadvantages include the potential for disease transmission and prolonged graft healing. Presented in this article are 2 techniques used at the authors' institution for primary ACL reconstruction with allograft. With the proper indications, knowledge of graft preparation and handling, and technique, allograft tissues in ACL reconstructions can provide the surgeon with clinical results equal to those of autograft reconstructions.

Allograft usage for cruciate ligament reconstruction has gained in popularity. Many techniques are described for posterior cruciate reconstruction with both autograft and allograft tendons. Achilles tendon allograft is a versatile and effective graft that can be used for a transtibial, double femoral bundle posterior cruciate reconstruction.

Meniscal allograft transplantation has emerged as a treatment option for selected meniscus-deficient patients to restore normal meniscal function and forestall progressive joint degeneration. Contraindications include diffuse subchondral bone exposure, axial malalignment, and instability. However, a knee may be rendered suitable for meniscus transplantation if combined with chondral resurfacing, osteotomy, and/or ligament reconstruction. Although numerous studies have reported improved clinical outcomes with meniscal allograft transplantation, high-quality studies with control groups are lacking in the literature. This article describes the current indications, graft types and sizing, surgical techniques, and a review of the literature with a focus on the role of concomitant procedures.

The use of osteochondral allografts to treat focal osteochondral lesions continues to gain popularity, supported by long-term results. Clinicians must be knowledgeable concerning the possible risks of disease transmission, graft rejection, infection, and graft failure to advise the patient and obtain an informed consent. With advancing scientific and clinical research, future operative indications will likely continue to expand. A significant amount of literature regarding storage methods has recently been published; it is hoped that continued research will lead to techniques for prolonged graft storage to prevent availability concerns.

Injuries to the collateral ligaments of the knee are very common. Recognition of collateral ligament laxity is extremely important, especially when associated with a cruciate ligament injury. Reconstruction of the collaterals are necessary when addressing these combined instabilities.

Revision anterior cruciate ligament (ACL) reconstruction presents many technical considerations not seen in primary ACL reconstruction. A variety of allograft options are available for use during revision ACL reconstruction, including bone-patella tendon-bone, calcaneus-Achilles tendon, and all soft-tissue grafts. Anatomic double-bundle ACL technique improves knee kinematics and provides the rotatory stability necessary to return to ACL-dependent activities.

Allografts play a prominent role in sports medicine, and their usage has increased dramatically over the past few decades, but the role of allograft in the future of sports medicine largely depends on several factors: (1) the ability of the tissue banking industry to convince both surgeons and the general population that tissue procurement is safe and nearly disease-free, (2) the ability to sterilize tissue with minimal compromise to tissue integrity, (3) successful clinical outcomes with allograft, and (4) the advent of artificial scaffolds and ligaments that function as well.

THE CLINICS ARE NOW AVAILABLE ONLINE!

Access your subscription at:
www.theclinics.com

Foreword

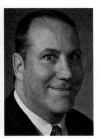

Mark D. Miller, MD
Consulting Editor

Whenever I discuss the possible use of allograft tissue with patients, they invariably ask where the tissue comes from. I usually explain to them that "it comes from someone who signs the back of their driver's license." This always gets the point across without stirring up too many gruesome images. The bigger concern to many patients these days is the recent press coverage about disease transmission and funeral home "donations."

I asked my good friend and former "fellow fellow" to spearhead an issue in *Clinics in Sports Medicine* on this important issue. He has assembled an impressive list of allograft experts to cover these topics. As alluded to in my opening paragraph, allograft safety is, and should be, the first topic for this issue. The topic that follows, tissue processing, is also an important consideration. We are aware from earlier work by Doug Jackson that allograft incorporation can be delayed when compared with autograft incorporation, and the third topic provides an update on that concern. What follows is an update on the allograft versus autograft debate. This is followed by a series of clinical scenarios for possible allograft use: anterior cruciate ligament, posterior cruciate ligament, meniscus, osteochondral grafts, collateral ligament reconstruction, and revision knee surgery.

The issue concludes with a thoughtful look into the future of allografts by Dr. Chris Harner, a mentor of both the guest editor and consulting editor for *Clinics*.

This is an important topic and has been well organized and thoughtfully put together by Dr. Johnson. He has always had an interest in this area, and his enthusiasm is evident in this masterfully edited edition.

Mark D. Miller, MD
Division of Sports Medicine
University of Virginia
400 Ray C. Hunt Drive, Suite 330
Charlottesville, VA 22908-0159, USA

E-mail address:
mdm3p@virginia.edu (M.D. Miller)

Clin Sports Med 28 (2009) xi
doi:10.1016/j.csm.2009.01.001
0278-5919/09/$ – see front matter © 2009 Elsevier Inc. All rights reserved.
sportsmed.theclinics.com

Preface

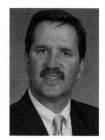

Darren L. Johnson, MD
Guest Editor

This issue is dedicated to the use of allograft tissue in knee surgery. During the last 20 to 30 years, the use of allograft tissue has increased exponentially, particularly as it relates to the field of sports medicine and knee surgery in the athletically active. Many high school and collegiate athletes have recovered from serious knee injuries and returned to the playing field because of our ability to use allograft tissue for replacement substitutes in complex knee problems. Along with this tremendous increase in the use of allograft tissue, a number of concerning issues have been brought to the forefront for discussion as well as to stimulate future research endeavors. I have asked national leaders within the knee surgery community to assist with this issue and its discussion. The table of contents is an outstanding one. I hope you will find it as enjoyable to read and learn from as I have in serving as the guest editor with these fine contributors.

I have asked Dr. Thomas Vangsness from the University of Southern California to update us on the safety and preparation of allograft tissue. Over the last 10 years, drastic improvements have been made to ensure the safety of allograft tissue with respect to not only the prevention of bacterial infection but also the transmission of viruses that could even be fatal in extreme, unlikely circumstances. Dr. Fred Azar from the Campbell Clinic has provided an outstanding review of the proprietary techniques used for tissue processing and the role of secondary sterilization techniques for allograft tissue. Many of these techniques are proprietary in nature, with specific details of that process lacking from many tissue banks. We still have much to learn about the role they play with respect to the biological incorporation process of the allograft and the eventual outcome of the surgical procedure. Future studies to define these proprietary techniques in an animal model are required and desperately needed.

I have asked Dr. David McAllister from the University of California, Los Angeles, to discuss the exact biology of allograft incorporation. Many of our studies have shown us that it appears to be "different" and somewhat delayed compared with the incorporation of autogenous tissue. It is important to many of us who use allograft tissue to understand fully what those differences are and, more importantly, how we might rehabilitate a patient differently who undergoes allograft versus autograft anterior cruciate

Clin Sports Med 28 (2009) xiii–xiv
doi:10.1016/j.csm.2008.11.001
0278-5919/08/$ – see front matter © 2009 Elsevier Inc. All rights reserved.

sportsmed.theclinics.com

ligament (ACL) surgery. If the biological incorporation is different between the 2, we may have to rehabilitate them differently for optimal outcome.

Dr. Ned Amendola from the University of Iowa has updated us in 2009 about what we really know when comparing allograft tissue to autograft tissue in cruciate ligament surgery. Although very few high-quality level 1 studies have been completed comparing the 2, Dr. Amendola has done an admirable job in presenting the facts as they stand in 2009. Dr. Peter Indelicato from the University of Florida has discussed his rationale for the use of Achilles tendon allograft tissue in primary ACL reconstruction in the athletically active. He has had outstanding success with his patients over the last 10 years.

Dr. Gene Barrett from Jackson, Mississippi, has discussed his use of allograft tissue in reconstruction of posterior cruciate ligament.

Dr. Scott Rodeo from the Hospital for Special Surgery has provided us with an outstanding review and update of the current concepts of meniscal allografts in 2009. Dr. Christian Lattermann from the University of Kentucky has discussed the use of osteochondral allografts and the state of the art in 2009.

I have asked Dr. Walt Shelton from Jackson, Mississippi, to share with us his rationale for the use of allograft tissue in collateral ligament augmentation and reconstruction in the multiple-ligament-injured knee.

I have written of my own experience in using Achilles tendon allograft tissue in revision anatomic double-bundle ACL surgery in the Bluegrass experience from the University of Kentucky. Finally, Dr. Chris Harner from the University of Pittsburgh, who has an outstanding wealth of knowledge and experience with the use of autograft tissue, has given us his views on what he sees as the future role of allografts in sports medicine as it relates to knee surgery.

I want to personally thank the contributors for devoting their time and energy to this valuable educational effort. It is an honor to have worked with them in making this issue a tremendous success. I hope you find this issue of *Clinics in Sports Medicine* informative, interesting, and, most importantly, an asset to the care of the patients whom we are privileged to care for. It has been an honor and pleasure to serve as the guest editor for this informative issue. We should always remember that ultimately it is we as surgeons who are the "tissue bankers" for the patient. When considering and using allograft tissue, safety of use is the number 1 priority. We as surgeons must not take that responsibility lightly.

Darren L. Johnson, MD
Department of Orthopaedic Surgery
University of Kentucky
740 South Limestone
Suite K415 Kentucky Clinic
Lexington, KY 40536, USA

E-mail address:
dljohns@uky.edu (D.L. Johnson)

Current Safety Sterilization and Tissue Banking Issues for Soft Tissue Allografts

C. Thomas Vangsness, Jr., MD*, Ryan D. Dellamaggiora, MD

KEYWORDS

• Allograft • Tissue bank • Processing • Graft • Safety

The number of recent grafts harvested and *implanted* in the United States has steadily increased. According to the American Association of Tissue Banks (AATB), the number of grafts distributed increased from 500,000 in 1998 to 1,300,000 in 2003.[1] This trend has been seen in other countries as well.[2–4] Although they are used in other specialties, allografts are used predominantly in orthopedic sports medicine and reconstructive procedures. Orthopedic surgeons more often make daily decisions on the use and implantation of these tissue grafts. Many surgeons do not have a great understanding about allograft tissue and tissue banking. According to a recent survey by the American Orthopaedic Society for Sports Medicine (AOSSM), over 85% reported using allografts and over half of those surveyed did not know whether their grafts were sterilized or the specific sterilization process used.[5,6]

The public is concerned regarding the safety of allografts and transmission of disease.[7] As complications from allograft contamination have occurred, so has oversight from government agencies such as the Food and Drug Administration (FDA) and Centers for Disease Control and Prevention (CDC).

REGULATION ISSUES

Oversight of tissue processors is mandated by state and federal regulations and has greatly improved in the last decade. Human cells or tissues intended for another human recipient are classified as "human cell, tissue, and cellular and tissue-based products" (HCT/P). The federal code established in 2004 mandated the FDA Center for Biologics Evaluation and Research (CBER) to regulate HCT/P.[8] These regulations required tissue banks to register and list their HCT/P with the FDA, to screen and test

---

Department of Orthopaedic Surgery, University of Southern California, Keck School of Medicine, Healthcare Consultation Center, 1520 San Pablo Street, Suite 2000, Los Angeles, CA 90033 4608, USA
* Corresponding author.
E-mail address: vangsnes@usc.edu (C.T. Vangsness).

Clin Sports Med 28 (2009) 183–189
doi:10.1016/j.csm.2008.10.008
0278-5919/08/$ – see front matter © 2009 Elsevier Inc. All rights reserved.

donors to reduce the transmission of communicable diseases, and to keep detailed records documenting the type of tissue processed, tests performed, results, and destination of the tissue.

Federal and state governments are not the only entities who have oversight of the tissue banks. The Joint Commission (JC), formerly known as the Joint Commission on Accreditation of Healthcare Organizations (JCAHO), is a regulatory entity independent of the FDA. In 2007, the JC released the latest version of Tissue Storage and Issuance Standards.[9] These standards apply to implantable and transplantable products that are human or cellular based. The JC requires hospitals, critical access hospitals, ambulatory office-based surgery, and outpatient centers to develop procedures to address the critical areas of tissue recovery and storage, record-keeping and tracking, and adverse events/infection follow-up. These written procedures are required to describe protocols for tissue ordering, receipt, temperature-monitored storage, tissue handling, preparation for use, tracking the graft from receipt to implantation, and investigation/reporting of adverse events or possible infections. According to these guidelines, hospitals and surgery centers should be able to trace any tissue bidirectionally to report potential disease transmission to the recipient when notified by the tissue bank as well as report to the donor facility any adverse reactions. This improves record-keeping and adverse event monitoring. They have power of accreditation over hospitals and tissue banks, which, without these entities, would have difficulty billing state and private insurance companies, providing further new quality controls for current allograft tissue.

An organization critical to the regulation of tissue banks is the AATB. Founded in 1976, the AATB is a nonprofit organization to spread voluntary safety standards and ensure that human tissues intended for transplantation are safe and free of infectious disease, are of uniform high quality, and are available in quantities sufficient to meet national needs.

The AATB first published its Standard for Tissue Banking in 1984. Since then, it has been updated and revised, with the 12th edition released in 2008.[10] Two years after the release of the Standard for Tissue Banking, the AATB began an accreditation program for institutions. This was followed 2 years later by a certification program for individuals. Accreditation is renewed every 3 years and is based on compliance with its standards. In addition, the AATB may perform surprise inspections to ensure compliance.[11]

The AATB standards are stringent. Specifically, the AATB required nucleic acid testing (NAT) for human immunodeficiency virus (HIV) and hepatitis C virus (HCV) in March 2005. NAT reduces the window period, which is the time between infection and when the virus is detectable. The FDA later required this testing in August 2007.

The AATB is also strict regarding culture results. It requires that any processed allograft that tests positive for *Clostridium* or *Streptococcus pyogenes* be discarded.[6,12] Furthermore, the AATB requires that a graft with positive final culture be discarded if there is no validated protocol to eliminate the identified organism.

Currently, the AATB has 106 accredited tissue banks, and it has been estimated that AATB-accredited tissue banks distribute 90% of musculoskeletal tissues in the United States.[12] Membership in the AATB is voluntary, and the AATB does not have any formal disciplinary powers outside of restriction or removal of AATB accreditation. The "committee on biological implants tissue work group" of the American Academy of Orthopaedic Surgeons have urged the orthopedic surgeons to work with AATB tissue banks and "know their tissue banker."[13] Other authors have stated that a tissue bank not accredited by the AATB should be "a red flag"[14] with respect to quality.

INFECTION/DISEASE TRANSMISSION ISSUES

Over 10 million grafts have been implanted in the past 20 years, and relatively few incidents of disease transmission have been reported. Based on reports in the literature, the incidence of infections is estimated to be 0.02% from around 20,000 transplants a year and 0.0004% from around 900,000 allografts per year.[15] A survey performed by the AATB reported the incidence of allograft-related infection for the years 2003-2004. There were 192 reports of suspected allograft infections overall in 1.35 million grafts for an incidence of 0.014%. Forty-two percent of these allografts were soft tissue grafts, and 59% of these grafts involved orthopedic/sports medicine procedures. During this period, there were only 2 probable/confirmed allograft-related infections for an incidence of 0.00015%.[15] This is compared with a postoperative infection rate of 0.6% to 2%.[16]

PROCUREMENT AND PROCESSING

There are several critical steps taken during allograft procurement and processing to reduce the risk of transmission. These steps include donor screening, tissue procurement, tissue processing, and packaging/final sterilization. It is important to discuss the effects that these different tissue processing/sterilization techniques have on the graft properties.

Disease transmission with allograft transplants is possible from 2 main sources: an infected donor and contamination from tissue processing and packaging. To prevent transmission, Good Tissue Practices use several steps to reduce infections from allografts. The first is to prevent infected tissue from entering the donation pool. This is done by screening and donor selection. This process is further refined by cultures taken from the tissues themselves or their liquid environment. The next step is to prevent contamination. This is completed by performing the procurement in a timely fashion under aseptic conditions. The third step is to reduce or eliminate infecting agents. Newer processing techniques promise improved allograft safety without graft compromise. This is achieved during tissue processing as well as final sterilization.

One of the primary ways to prevent disease transmission by allograft transplantation is appropriate donor selection.[10,17] The most important step is a careful history and identification of risk factors for infectious diseases. This should also include a careful review of the medical history from different sources, including surviving family members, hospitals, clinics, and private doctor's offices. Other records such as blood donation history or autopsy records can also be obtained. The next step in donor screening is testing for an active infection. There are limitations of tests that rely on the presence of antibodies or antigens, such that there is a window period where the donor is actively infected but exhibits no detectable immunologic response. NAT reduces the window period from 22 days (HIV) and 70 days (HCV) to 7 days.[13] With current screening and testing protocols, the estimated risk of implanting tissue from an HIV-infected donor is 1 in 173,000 to 1 in 1 million. The estimated risk of implanting tissue from an HCV-infected donor is 1 in 421,000.[18] The risk of contracting hepatitis is much higher than the risk of HIV. The estimated prevalence of 1.2 million with hepatitis B and 3.2 million with HCV[19] is responsible for the increased risk. The incidence of HCV in the general population is 1.8%, and many of these patients do not know that they are carriers. Furthermore, 50% of carriers have no history of hepatitis or even know that they are seropositive.[20] The actual numbers of potential tissue donors that are infected with these viruses are unknown, and these numbers do not take into account the processing steps to reduce the risk of disease transmission.

Emerging pathogens have raised concern regarding the safety of allografts. There are very few data regarding the potential threat from the West Nile virus and the severe acute respiratory syndrome (SARS) coronavirus. Furthermore, there is no current screening test for prior diseases associated with spongiform encephalopathies. The risk of acquiring these diseases from a tissue allograft is unknown but is likely to be rare as is the overall incidence of these diseases in the general population.

Tissue recovery is the next step in minimizing the potential for disease transmission. According to the CDC, allograft tissue should not be considered sterile and the health care provider should be informed of the possible risk for bacterial infection.[21] Recovery of tissue is performed under aseptic conditions, under standard sterile operating room techniques, yet contamination can be introduced by the human handling the tissues. Time to harvest is also critical to reduce the risk of infection; according to AATB guidelines, tissue procurement must take place within 24 hours of asystole if the body is cooled or 15 hours if the body is not cooled.[12] Contamination has been documented from the breakdown of the donor's gastrointestinal or respiratory systems, and recovering tissue after this period has resulted in contamination and implanted infections.[11,22]

As each tissue is procured, it is cultured, wrapped, labeled, and sealed in dedicated containers at wet ice temperatures. Surface swab cultures are performed to evaluate for the presence of bacteria and fungi; they are not used to establish sterility but to monitor previously validated sterilizing processes. Studies have shown that surface swab cultures are only 78% to 92% sensitive.[23]

STERILIZATION ISSUES

After the tissues are procured, they must be processed and secondarily sterilized. Many tissue banks have their own proprietary sterilization technique. Ideally, a sterilization process should eliminate any microorganisms while maintaining the mechanical and biological characteristics of the allograft. Furthermore, any sterilization reagent used should permeate the tissue and be safely removed from the tissue without residue.

Sterilization is expressed as a mathematical probability of relative risk. The FDA requires a sterility assurance level (SAL) of 10^{-3} for implantation of a medical device. This means that there is a 1 in 1000 probability that a viable microbe exists in or on the implantable device. This is the acceptable level of SAL for HCT/Ps (human tissues). Many tissue banks, however, are applying AATB sterility standards required for medical devices at a level of SAL of 10^{-6}.

There are many different tissue processing methods used by tissue banks. Several tissue banks have a proprietary sterilizing method to process tissues, which must be validated and documented on site for any surprise inspection by the FDA regulators. **Table 1** outlines many of the processes used by major tissue banks.

Some tissue banks use gamma radiation to sterilize their products after packaging. This is referred to as terminal sterilization. Low-dose (<2 Mrad) gamma radiation is documented to be effective at sterilization, but studies have also shown that it generates free radicals that can adversely affect the structure of collagen and ultimately the mechanical properties of the graft. Higher radiation levels (>2 Mrad) have demonstrated biomechanical weakening of the collagen tissues.[24] Historically, ethylene oxide (ETO) gas was used for terminal sterilization, but its use was discontinued because of documented patient tissue reactions with ETO-treated grafts.[22]

At this time, there is no one ideal sterilization technique for soft tissue allografts. The FDA does not specify which process or technique should be used. The FDA only

Table 1	
Tissue banks and tissue-processing techniques	
Tissue bank	**Sterilization method**
AlloSource	SterileR validated bioburden reduction cleansing system followed by low-dose terminal irradiation to provide SAL 10^{-6}. Package is labeled "sterile."
Bone Bank Allografts	GraftCleanse: proprietary blend of cleansing agents used to reduce bioburden and provide aesthetic white appearance. GraftCleanse: terminal low-dose gamma irradiation achieves package sterility.
Community Tissue Services (CTS)	Musculoskeletal grafts are soaked and rinsed in antibiotics, hydrogen peroxide, alcohol, sterile water, and AlloWash solutions. Low-dose terminal gamma irradiation is used to eliminate most bacteria.
LifeNet	AlloWash XG: rigorous cleansing removes blood elements followed by decontamination and a scrubbing regimen to eliminate bacteria and viruses. Tissue is terminally irradiated at a low dose to reach SAL 10^{-6} and is labeled "sterile."
Musculoskeletal Tissue Foundation (MTF)	MTF processes soft tissue allografts aseptically and treats the grafts with an antibiotic cocktail of gentamicin, amphotericin B, and imipenem and cilastatin sodium (Primaxin). Some incoming tissue is pretreated with low-dose gamma irradiation to reduce bioburden. No terminal irradiation used.
OsteoTech	OsteoTech processes allograft tissue using aseptic technique in class 100 clean rooms. Isolators are used to prevent cross-contamination.
RTI Biologics, Inc.	BioCleanse: an automated chemical sterilization process that is validated to remove blood, marrow, and lipids and eliminate bacteria, fungi, spores, and viruses while maintaining biomechanical integrity and biocompatibility. No preprocessing or terminal irradiation is used on sports medicine allografts. All tissues reach SAL 10^{-6} post-BioCleanse.
Tissue Banks International (TBI)	Clearant Process: pathogen inactivation process involving high-dose gamma irradiation at (5.0 Mrad) combined with radioprotectant that sterilizes tissue in the final packaging, significantly inactivates infectious agents, and maintains the function of the allograft. Process yields SAL 10^{-6} and package is labeled "sterile."

requires that claims of sterility be documented and validated. The 2002 guidelines state that these representations are subject to scrutiny by the FDA. Tissue studies are often performed on tissue immersed in the pathogen of interest and not from systemically infected donors. This is not the ideal infection model.

STORAGE OF ALLOGRAFT TISSUES

After procuring, processing, and packaging, allograft tissues are stored frozen. According to AATB guidelines, musculoskeletal tissues should be stored at $-40°$C or colder and can be held for up to 5 years.[10] A temperature range of $-20°$C to $-40°$C is thought to be a more short-term storage condition and safe for up to 6 months. When shipped between supplier and end user, tissue should be kept on dry ice.[12]

DISCUSSION

Allograft implantation in orthopedic procedures has increased steadily over the last decade. Patient infections and widespread media coverage have raised concern regarding the safety and efficacy of the allografts. Tissue banks, government agencies, and non-profit organizations have undergone multilevel changes to reduce the risk of disease transmission. Safely procuring and processing the grafts and thorough screening of donors have improved the quality of the allograft pool and decreased the risk of disease transmission. The regulatory agencies hope to ensure graft safety through improved regulation and standardized treatment methods. Finally, improved communication with a unique identification for each graft and donor leads to more efficient future monitoring and detection of infections and perhaps prevention of implantation of suspected tissues. All these steps make the clinical use of musculoskeletal allografts the safest it has ever been for the patient.

As newer methods of sterilization are developed, further biologic and biomechanical tests need to be performed. As tissue banks state claims of sterility and biomechanical properties, these statements should be independently evaluated. Oversight by governing bodies should provide monitoring and long-term follow-up of these new processes. As recommended by the American Academy of Orthopaedic Surgeons, surgeons need to be familiar with the tissue bank they work with and how their grafts are processed. Tissue banks and the processing of graft tissues still face challenges. Emerging diseases and pathogens reveal the need for more sensitive testing. Ultimately, the patients will continue to have improved tissue safety now and in the future.

REFERENCES

1. Centers for Disease Control and Prevention. About tissue transplants. Available at: http://www.cdc.gov/ncidod/dhqp/tissueTransplantsFAQ.html. Accessed September 1, 2008.
2. Bohatyrewicz A, Bohatyrewicz R, Dobiecki K, et al. Is retrieval of bone material from multiorgan donors effective enough to cover demand for biostatic bone tissue grafts in Poland? Transplant Proc 2006;38(1):297–300.
3. Lakey JR, Mirbolooki M, Rogers C, et al. Supply of human allograft tissue in Canada. Cell Tissue Bank 2007;8(2):135–50 [Epub 2006 Jun 28].
4. Galvan R, Briseno R, Alvarez E, et al. Tissue banking in Mexico. Cell Tissue Bank 2006;7(3):215–20.
5. 2006 AOSSM orthopaedic surgical procedure survey on allografts. Naperville (IL): Leever Research Services; 2006.
6. McAllister DR, Joyce MJ, Mann BJ, et al. Allograft update—the current status of tissue regulation, procurement, processing, and sterilization. Am J Sports Med 2007;35:2148–58.
7. MSNBC. Vote: how do you feel about tissue donation?. Available at: http://msnbc.msn.com/id/14520590. Updated August 28, 2006.
8. US Food and Drug Administration. Current good tissue practice for human cell, tissue, and cellular and tissue-based product establishments: inspection and enforcement; final rule 21 CFR parts 16, 1270, and 1271 (D, E, E) 69 fed reg: 16–611-68688. Available at: http://www.fda.gov/cber/tiss.htm. Accessed September 19, 2008.
9. Joint Commission. New standards PC.17.10, PC.17.20, and PC.17.30. Available at: http://www.jointcommission.org/. Accessed July 1, 2005.
10. Standards for tissue banking. 12th edition. McLean (VA): American Association of Tissue Banks; 2007. Available at: http://www.aatb.org. Accessed January 21, 2009.

11. Vangsness CT Jr, Garcia IA, Mills CR, et al. Allograft transplantation in the knee: tissue regulation, procurement, processing, and sterilization. Am J Sports Med 2003;31:474–81.
12. The American Association of Tissue Banks. Available at: http://www.aatb.org. Accessed September 23, 2008.
13. American Academy of Orthopaedic Surgeons. American Academy of Orthopaedic Surgeons advisory statement #1011: use of musculoskeletal tissue allografts. Available at: http://www.aaos.org/about/papers/advistmt/1011.asp. Accessed January 1, 2009.
14. Branam BR, Johnson DL. Allografts in knee surgery. Orthopedics 2007;30(11): 925–9.
15. Workshop on preventing organ and tissue allograft–transmitted infection: priorities for public health intervention June 2–3, 2005; Atlanta (GA).
16. NNIS System, Division of Healthcare Quality Promotion, National Center for Infectious Diseases, CDC, Public Health Service, US Dept. of Health and Human Services, Atlanta (GA); National Nosocomial Infections Surveillance (NNIS) System Reports, data summary from January 1992 through June 2004, issued October 2004.
17. Gocke DJ. Tissue donor selection and safety. Clin Orthop Relat Res 2005 Jun;(435):17–21.
18. Zou S, Dodd RY, Stramer SL, et al. Probability of viremia with HBV, HCV, HIV, and HTLV among tissue donors in the United States. N Engl J Med 2004;351:751–9.
19. Centers for Disease Control and Prevention. Viral hepatitis: statistics and surveillance. Available at: http://www.cdc.gov/hepatitis/Statistics.htm. Accessed September 23, 2008.
20. Centers for Disease Control and Prevention. Recommendations for prevention and control of hepatitis C virus (HCV) infection and HCV-related chronic disease. MMWR Recomm Rep 1998;47(RR-19):1–39.
21. Centers for Disease Control and Prevention. Update: allograft-associated bacterial infections—United States, 2002. MMWR Morb Mortal Wkly Rep 2002;51: 207–10.
22. Vangsness CT Jr, Wagner PP, Moore TM, et al. Overview of safety issues concerning the preparation and processing of soft-tissue allografts. Arthroscopy 2006; 22(12):1351–8.
23. Veen MR, Bloem RM, Petit PL. Sensitivity and negative predictive value of swab cultures in musculoskeletal allograft procurement. Clin Orthop 1994;300:259–63.
24. Fideler BM, Vangsness CT Jr, Moore T, et al. Effects of gamma irradiation on the human immunodeficiency virus: a study in frozen human bone-patellar ligament-bone grafts obtained from infected cadavers. J Bone Joint Surg Am 1994;76: 1032–5.

Tissue Processing: Role of Secondary Sterilization Techniques

Frederick M. Azar, MD

KEYWORDS

• Allograft • Musculoskeletal • Sterilization

The use of allografts in sports medicine surgery has been steadily increasing over the past 10 to 15 years as long-term reports have shown that results with musculoskeletal allografts approach those with autografts.[1–4] The use of musculoskeletal allografts from the American Association of Tissue Banks (AATB) accredited tissue banks increased from 337,338 in 1996 to 1,279,000 in 2003 (**Table 1**).[5] Each year approximately 1.5 million bone and tissue allografts are implanted in the United States, of which approximately 10% are soft-tissue grafts, most commonly bone-patellar tendon-bone (BPTB), Achilles tendon (**Fig. 1**), fascia lata, anterior and posterior tibial tendon (**Fig. 2**), quadriceps and hamstring tendon, and menisci.[6,7] A 2006 member survey by the American Orthopaedic Society for Sports Medicine (AOSSM) indicated that 86% used allografts in knee reconstructive procedures;[8,9] however, despite this widespread use, a substantial number of surgeons expressed concerns about the risk of disease transmission and infection with allografts. A number of advantages of allografts over autografts have been cited, including no donor-site morbidity, shorter operative time, smaller incisions, and greater availability, but all of these have been overshadowed by the most frequently cited disadvantage: risk of disease transmission.[10–12] Recent reports of serious infections associated with allografts have heightened these concerns.[13–15] Of 26 bacterial infections associated with allografts reported to the Centers for Disease Control and Prevention (CDC), 70% were in patients who had anterior cruciate ligament (ACL) reconstructions.[13,14] A 2004 report[16] indicated that of the 875,000 musculoskeletal allografts distributed in 2001, clostridium infections occurred in 0.12% of all sports medicine tissues (tendons, menisci, and femoral condyles).

University of Tennessee-Campbell Clinic Department of Orthopaedic Surgery, 1211 Union Avenue, Suite 520, Memphis, TN 38104, USA
E-mail address: fazar@campbellclinic.com

Clin Sports Med 28 (2009) 191–201
doi:10.1016/j.csm.2008.10.003   **sportsmed.theclinics.com**
0278-5919/08/$ – see front matter © 2009 Elsevier Inc. All rights reserved.

Table 1		
Donors and distribution from AATB-accredited tissue banks		
Year	No. of Donors	Musculoskeletal Tissue Allografts Distributed
1996	17,010	337,338
2001	20,490	710,064
2003	23,295	1,279,000

Data from Vangsness CT Jr. How safe are soft-tissue allografts? AAOS Now, August 2007. Available at: http://www.aaos.org/news/bulletin/aug07/clinical1.asp.

RISK OF DISEASE TRANSMISSION FROM MUSCULOSKELETAL ALLOGRAFTS

Donor screening and testing (**Table 2**) can reduce the possibility of disease transmission, but a "window" period still exists during which a donor with an active viral infection may not have any detectable viral antibodies or antigens.[17] With nucleic acid testing (NAT), this window is approximately 7 days for human immunodeficiency virus (HIV) and hepatitis-C virus (HCV) and about 8 days for hepatitis-B virus (HBV).[18] Currently, the risk of transplanting tissue from an HIV-infected donor is estimated to be 1 in 1.6 million.[11,19–21] Because of the greater prevalence of hepatitis in the general population, estimated to be 1.2 million infected with HBV and 3.9 million with HCV,[17] the risk of the transmission of HBV or HCV is greater than that of HIV. The risk of contracting HCV from unprocessed tissue that is NAT HCV negative is estimated to be 1 in 421,000.[21] McAllister and colleagues[9] noted that the current risk of an allograft-transmitted infection appears to be much less than the overall risk of perioperative nosocomial infection.

More recently, emerging pathogens have become a concern in the use of allograft material. Little information exists about the potential threat from such entities as West Nile virus, severe acute respiratory syndrome (SARS) coronavirus, and prion disease associated with transmissible spongiform encephalopathies such as Creutzfeldt-Jakob disease (CJD) and its variants. Between 1985 and 2002, 97 occurrences of CJD were reported in Japanese patients who had received dura mater allografts; the rate of infection declined after improved processing procedures were introduced in 1987.[22] No prion-disease transmission has been reported in association with musculoskeletal allografts, and the risk of acquiring these diseases as the result of

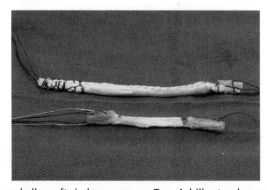

Fig. 1. Commonly used allografts in knee surgery. Top, Achilles tendon graft used for reconstruction of the posterior cruciate ligament. Bottom, Bone-patellar tendon-bone graft used for reconstruction of the anterior cruciate ligament.

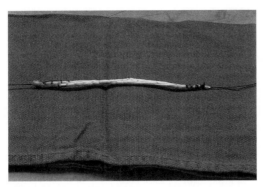

Fig. 2. Tibialis allograft.

Table 2
Process of allograft procurement, sterilization, and storage

Donor screening	Precluded by history of autoimmune disease
	Ingestion or exposure to toxic substances
	Rheumatoid arthritis
	Systemic lupus erythematosus
	Polyarteritis nodosa
	Sarcoidosis
	Clinically significant bone disease
	Blood testing must be negative for antibodies to HIV
	Nucleic acid test (NAT) for HIV-1
	Hepatitis B surface antigen
	Total antibody to hepatitis B core antigen,
	Antibodies to hepatitis C virus (HCV)
	NAT for HCV
	Antibodies to human T-lymphotropic virus
	Syphilis
Tissue harvest	Within 24 h of death if body cooled
	Within 15 h of death if body not cooled
	Aseptic technique
	Tissue cultured before processing
Disinfection: removal of contaminants	Antibiotic soaks
Secondary sterilization: destruction of all life forms	Ethyl oxide, other chemical sterilants
	Gamma/electron-beam irradiation
	Proprietary protocols (ie, Allowash, BioClense, Clearant)
Storage	Fresh allograft (use within 24 d)
	Fresh-freezing (3–5 y)
	Cryopreservation (up to 10 y)
	Lypophilization (3–5 y at room temperature)

a musculoskeletal allograft is unknown, although it is likely extremely low because of the rarity of these diseases in the general population.[9]

OVERSIGHT OF PREPARATION OF MUSCULOSKELETAL ALLOGRAFTS

In the United States,oversight of tissue banks takes place at 3 levels: the American Association of Tissue Banks (AATB), the Food and Drug Administration (FDA), and state agencies.[6] The AATB has developed standards for tissue banking, and it accredits tissue banks but has no power to shut down a tissue bank, fine or imprison its operators, or order the retention or destruction of tissue that does not comply with minimal requirements.[6] The FDA does have that power, but one of their limitations is that registration of tissue banks has not been required, making it difficult for the FDA to identify and inspect such entities.[23,24] Only a small percentage of tissue banks are AATB-accredited, and few states require tissue banks to be licensed. In 2005, the FDA set up 3 new regulations for entities involved in human tissue products: "registration" rules for tissue banking institutions, "donor eligibility" rules that provide criteria for donor screening and selection, and "current good tissue practices" rules that concern tissue procurement, processing, and distribution.[25] Currently, there is more federal oversight of tissue banks and improved donor screening and testing techniques, including the use of NAT. In the United States, all establishments that collect, process, or handle human cells, tissues, and cellular or tissue-based products must now register with the FDA.

DECREASING THE RISK OF DISEASE TRANSMISSION BY MUSCULOSKELETAL ALLOGRAFTS

The FDA does not require that tissues undergo sterilization nor does it require that recovery and processing of tissues be done in an aseptic manner, both of which are essential to improving allograft safety.[24] Sterilization of musculoskeletal tissues has several inherent problems: the biomechanical integrity of the tissue can be substantially altered by heat and irradiation, not all sterilizing agents have adequate tissue penetration, and musculoskeletal tissues are often contaminated with a large number of organisms.

Aseptic Procurement

Aseptic procurement is a fairly standardized procedure in which standard sterile operating room techniques are used, including using gowns, gloves, and sterile instruments. Aseptically processed tissues, however, should not be considered sterile.[26] Contamination from health care personnel or from the donor (gastrointestinal or respiratory tract) may not be eliminated or even adequately reduced by soaking in antibiotic solution, as is done in most tissue banks to reduce the surface contamination (bioburden) of the allograft tissue. Although culturing of allograft tissue is commonly done to check for the presence of bacteria and fungi after soaking, studies have shown that cultures are, at best, only 78% to 92% sensitive.[27]

Disinfection and Secondary Sterilization

Disinfection—removal of contaminants from the tissue—should not be mistaken for sterilization—destruction of all forms of life, especially microorganisms. Sterility is expressed as a mathematic probability of relative risk. The FDA considers a sterility assurance level (SAL) of 10^{-3} (1 in 1,000 chance that a nonviral viable microbe exists) adequate for implantable biologic medical devices.[24] The AATB requires an SAL of 10^{-6} (less than a 1 in 1,000,000 possibility of a contaminating organism) for tissue bank allografts.[28] Unlike surgical instruments and equipment, it is practically impossible to absolutely sterilize human tissue without compromising the biomechanical properties or biocompatibility of these tissues. For example, heat and high doses of radiation (>3.0 Mrad) can effectively provide an SAL of 10^{-6}, but both can weaken the collagen structure of the allograft.[29,30]

Chemical sterilization

Chemical sterilization agents have included peracetic acid (PAA), ethylene oxide, hydrogen peroxide, supercritical carbon dioxide, beta-propiolactone, and glutaraldehyde; the last 2 are no longer used because of their toxicity, and the others are generally used in combination with other methods of sterilization.

Ethylene oxide, commonly used for sterilizing medical devices, was one of the first methods used to sterilize allografts.[31] Chemical residues left by the sterilization process, however, were suggested to cause intra-articular reactions with chronic synovitis, graft failure, and bone dissolution.[32,33] Ethylene oxide has been reported to have some carcinogenic effects in workers exposed to it,[34] but there is no evidence that allografts sterilized with ethylene oxide have induced cancer.[20] In patellar tendon grafts, ethylene oxide can cause a foreign body reaction that results in dissolution of the graft,[32,33,35] termed the "applesauce reaction" by Arnoczky because of the appearance of the dissolved graft.[36] This sterilization method is rarely used today.

PAA has been used since the early 1980s, mainly to sterilize bone allografts. Several preliminary in vitro studies suggested that it produced no adverse effects on the structural and mechanical properties of treated bone grafts.[37,38] Analyses of the mechanical function of BPTB grafts in vitro revealed no adverse effects of PAA sterilization compared with unsterilized grafts.[39] A more recent study,[40] however, found in a goat model that PAA sterilization delayed or partially inhibited the biological remodeling of PAA grafts, leading to impaired functional knee stability and reduced structural properties of the graft during subsequent healing up to 3 months. The authors recommend caution when considering PAA-sterilized allografts for ACL reconstruction.

Radiation sterilization

Gamma irradiation has been shown to be effective for sterilization of allograft tissues, killing bacteria at doses of 1.5 to 2.6 Mrad;[4] higher doses (>3.5 Mrad) are necessary to kill viruses.[29,30,41] Fideler and colleagues[29] found that some HIV-infected bone-tendon-bone allografts remained positive for the virus after 2.5 Mrad of irradiation and recommended that grafts be exposed to levels as high as 3.6 to 4 Mrad. Heat and high doses of radiation (>3.0 Mrad) can produce an SAL of 10^{-6}, but such high doses substantially affect the biomechanical properties of allografts.[29,30,42,43]

The effects of lower levels of irradiation on allografts remain an area of controversy.[44,45] Schwartz and colleagues[45] confirmed in a goat model that 4.0 Mrad caused 30% and 21% reductions in stiffness and maximal force, respectively, at 6 months after implantation. Even low-dose irradiation (2 Mrad, 20 kGy) has been shown to diminish the strength and increase the cyclic elongation of BPTB allografts.[46] Balsly and colleagues,[47] however, tested bone grafts (dowel and iliac crest wedge grafts) and soft-tissue grafts (patellar, anterior tibial, and semitendinosus tendons and fascia lata) exposed to low-dose (18.3–21.8 kGy) or moderate-dose (24.0–28.5 kGy) gamma irradiation and found no statistically significant differences in mechanical strength or modulus of elasticity for any graft irradiated at low-dose compared with controls. Bone allografts and 2 of the soft-tissue allografts (anterior tibial and semitendinosus tendons) demonstrated strength and modulus of elasticity values similar to those of controls.

Electron-beam radiation has been used for sterilization, primarily of soft-tissue grafts, because of its lower penetrability (8 cm through the density of water) compared with gamma irradiation (30 cm through the density of water), which would be a problem with cortical bone allografts, which have a density of about twice that of water.[48,49] The advantage to electron-beam irradiation is higher processing speed—seconds, compared with hours for gamma irradiation. Although one biomechanical cadaver study of electron-beam radiation combined with tissue-protective measures (low temperature, carbon dioxide) concluded that the process did not impair the mechanical properties of BPTB grafts,[50] another determined that both gamma and electron-beam irradiation caused reductions in tensile strength, elastic modulus, strain, and toughness of rabbit tendons.[49] The decreases in strength and toughness were dose-dependent: the average loss of tensile strength was 36% with 25 kGy and 55% with 50 kGy irradiation compared with controls.

Because research has supported the hypothesis that gamma radiation-induced allograft damage is caused, in part, by free radical attack on the molecular structure of the collagen,[51,52] a number of radioprotectants have been used to eliminate or decrease the deleterious effects of irradiation. Grieb and colleagues[53] reported that a radioprotective "cocktail" solution, which included propylene glycol, dimethyl sulfoxide (DMSO), mannitol, and trehalose, was successful in protecting mechanical properties of human semitendinosus tendon at 50 kGy under regulated conditions. Akkus and colleagues[51] reported that the use of another free radical scavenger, thiourea, resulted in increased toughness at 36 kGy in bone allografts. Seto and colleagues[49] used crosslinkers, including 1-ethyl-3-(3-dimethylaminopropyl) carbodiimide (EDC) and glucose to add exogenous crosslinks to collagen and compared their effects to those of free radical scavengers (mannitol, ascorbate, and riboflavin) in rabbit tendons. Both treatments protected mechanical properties at 25 kGy, but at 50 kGy crosslinkers were superior. The strength, modulus of elasticity, toughness, and strain of glucose-treated tendon, either gamma or electron-beam irradiated at 25 kGy, were close to those of native tendon. Kattaya and colleagues[54] noted that along with the beneficial effects of radioprotectants there is also the potential of radioprotection of pathogenic organisms and that the ideal radioprotectant should protect graft integrity without compromising sterility.

Combined methods of sterilization

Combining lower doses of irradiation (1–3.5 Mrad, 10–35 kGy) with other processing techniques, such as antibiotic soaks, is probably the most commonly used method today.

Several companies have proprietary processes for sterilization that each claims will provide a disease-free graft. Cryolife, Inc. (Kennesaw, GA) uses a slow freezing process along with DMSO or glycerol for cryopreservation of grafts. After swab culturing and desiccation, the grafts are treated for an extended period of time with an antimicrobial solution. No secondary sterilization method is used.

BioCleanse (Regeneration Technologies, Inc., Alachua, FL) is a low-temperature chemical sterilization method that is claimed to penetrate the tissue and eliminate endogenous contamination. The process permeates the inner matrix of tissue with liquid sterilants, such as hydrogen peroxide and isopropyl alcohol, followed by pressure variations to drive the sterilants in and out of the tissue. Soft-tissue grafts (bone-tendon-bone, fascia, tendons, and menisci) are treated with this method. Studies have shown that the BioCleanse process does not appear to affect the mechanical properties of BPTB grafts[55] or anterior tibial tendon grafts.[56]

Allowash (Lifenet, Virginia Beach, VA) uses ultrasonics, centrifugation, and negative pressure in combination with reagents, including biologic detergents, alcohols, and hydrogen peroxide. This process claims to increase solubilization and remove lipids, blood, and marrow cells that can act as reservoirs for potential bacterial, fungal, and viral agents. BPTB allografts are terminally sterilized using 13 to 18 kGy of radiation.

The Tutoplast process (RTI Biologics, Alachua, FL) also uses an ultrasonic acetone bath to remove lipids, followed by a series of alternating hyperosmotic saline and deionized water baths to destroy bacteria. An oxidative treatment with hydrogen peroxide is then used to eliminate soluble proteins and destroy nonenveloped viruses and bacterial spores. A final acetone wash is done to ensure that any residual prions are removed and enveloped viruses are inactivated and to dehydrate the tissue; this is followed by vacuum extraction, which allows storage at room temperature. Terminal sterilization is done with low-dose gamma irradiation.

The Clearant Process (Clearant, Inc., Los Angeles, CA) treats tissue with high doses of radiation (50 kGy), which is 2 to 4 times the dose recommended to avoid tissue damage but claims to avoid this by freezing the sample, extracting the water, and adding stabilizers and free radical scavengers. After the tissue is frozen and the water extracted, DMSO and propylene glycol are added as pretreatment radioprotectants.[53]

NovaSterilis (Lansing, NY) developed a technique of sterilization that uses supercritical carbon dioxide at low temperatures and relatively low pressures to induce transient acidification, which is lethal to viruses and bacteria. Although tissue penetration appears to be good with this method, data concerning the effects on the mechanical properties of allografts are limited at this time.

The Musculoskeletal Transplant Foundation (MTF, Edison, NJ), a non-profit organization, also uses a series of chemicals, including nonionic detergents, hydrogen peroxide, and alcohol, to treat most cortical and cancellous grafts, without terminal sterilization with irradiation. This process has been demonstrated to maintain osteoconductivity for up to 1 hour; compressive strength, impact strength, and shear strength are reported to be unaffected by the cleaning procedure.[57] BPTB and other soft-tissue allografts are treated with an antibiotic "cocktail" of gentamicin, amphotericin B, and Primaxin (imipenem and cilastatin). The antibiotics are washed out at the completion of processing to nondetectable levels. Low-dose gamma irradiation (12–18 kGy) is used for tissue that is found to have a bioburden (the number of contaminating organisms on a given amount of material before sterilization) greater than what could be sterilized by the antibiotic cocktail.

STORAGE OF PROCESSED ALLOGRAFT TISSUE

Once the allograft tissue has been processed, it must be preserved and stored until needed. Articular cartilage allografts may be used as "fresh" grafts, within 24 days of donor death, but most other allograft tissue is fresh-frozen, freeze-dried, or cryopreserved.

Fresh-freezing or deep-freezing is the simplest and most widely used storage method for ligament and meniscal tissue. After sterile tissue harvest, the tissue is cultured and then frozen while serologic tests are done; the tissue is then soaked in an antibiotic solution, packaged, and frozen. The AATB requires storage at a temperature of at least -40°C, but most tissue banks keep allografts at -70°C to -80°C, which allows storage for 3 to 5 years;[4,20] at a temperature near -196°C, grafts can be preserved for as long as 10 years.[4]

Freeze-drying or lyophilization (residual moisture content of less than 5%) destroys all cells within the tissue but has the advantage of allowing vacuum-packed storage at room temperature for 3 to 5 years. This method is not often used for sports medicine procedures in the United States because the process can degrade the mechanical properties of soft-tissue allografts.[3] A disadvantage is the need for a minimum of 30 minutes of rehydration of the graft before use, especially if a bone block is attached to the soft tissue. Freeze-drying alters the material properties of collagen but has not been shown to have a clinical effect.[20] One study[58] noted a significant association between the failure of freeze-dried allografts used for ACL reconstruction and the time from procurement to implantation, suggesting that the shelf life of freeze-dried tissues is limited. Another study[59] found that the ultimate strength of cancellous bone was reduced by 19% and stiffness by 20% in rehydrated lypophilized grafts, suggesting that the mechanical properties of lypophilized BPTB grafts may be inferior to those of fresh-frozen allografts.

Cryopreservation is a process by which the tissue undergoes controlled-rate freezing to -135°C while cellular water is extracted by glycerol and DMSO. Packed in a cryoprotectant solution, the graft has a shelf life of 10 years, and up to 80% of cells can remain viable.[4,9,20]

SUMMARY

No sterilization techniques have been definitively proven to be more effective than others, and their biomechanical and biological effects on allograft tissue remain largely unknown. Despite recent highly publicized occurrences of infection from allografts, however, the current risk of an allograft infection appears to be much less than the risk of infection surrounding the surgical procedure itself.[5,9] Most of these incidents involved questionable practices, violations of FDA regulations, and even alleged illegal activities by recovery agents.[13,15,24] According to a report from the AATB covering data from 2003 and 2004, of 192 reports of suspected allograft-related infections, 42% involved soft-tissue grafts and 37% involved bone grafts, with an overall incidence of 0.014%; 59% involved orthopedic sports medicine procedures.[9] The American Academy of Orthopaedic Surgeons (AAOS) recommends that surgeons choose tissue provided by an AATB-member tissue bank and that they be familiar with the different sterilization processes used for allografts.[60,61] With appropriate donor screening, improved donor testing, including NAT, and adherence to AATB standards, the risk of disease transmission or infections can be eliminated or substantially decreased.

REFERENCES

1. Harner CD, Olson E, Irrgang JJ, et al. Allograft versus autograft anterior cruciate ligament reconstruction: 3- to 5-year outcome. Clin Orthop Relat Res 1996;324: 134–44.
2. Lephart SM, Kocher MS, Harner CD, et al. Quadriceps strength and functional capacity after anterior cruciate ligament reconstruction. Patellar tendon autograft versus allograft. Am J Sports Med 1993;21:738–43.
3. Saddemi SR, Frogameni AD, Fenton PJ, et al. Comparison of perioperative morbidity of anterior cruciate ligament autografts versus allografts. Arthroscopy 1993;9:519–24.
4. Shelton WR. Arthroscopic allograft surgery of the knee and shoulder: indications, techniques, and risks. Arthroscopy 2003;19(Suppl 1):67–9.
5. Vangsness CT Jr. How safe are soft-tissue allografts? AAOS Now August 2007; Available at: http://www.aaos.org/news/bulletin/aug07/clinical1.asp. Accessed July 25, 2008.

6. Saurez LS, Richmond JC. Overview of procurement, processing, and sterilization of soft tissue allografts for sports medicine. Sports Med Arthrosc 2007;15:106–13.
7. Robertson A. Current trends in the use of tendon allografts in orthopaedic surgery. J Bone Joint Surg Br 2006;88B:988–92.
8. 2006 AOSSM Orthopaedic Surgical Procedure Survey on Allografts. Napier (IL): Leever Research Services; 2006. Accessed July 25, 2008.
9. McAllister DR, Joyce MJ, Mann BJ, et al. Allograft update: the current status of tissue regulation, procurement, processing, and sterilization. Am J Sports Med 2007;35:2148–58.
10. Branam BR, Johnson DL. Allografts in knee surgery. Orthopedics 2007;30:925–9.
11. Rihn JA, Harner CD. The use of musculoskeletal allograft tissue in knee surgery. Arthroscopy 2003;19(Suppl 1):51–66.
12. Patel R, Trampuz A. Infections transmitted through musculoskeletal tissue allografts. N Engl J Med 2004;350:2544–6.
13. Centers for Disease Control and Prevention. Update: allograft associated bacterial infections-United States, 2002. MMWR Morb Mortal Wkly Rep 2002;51:207–10.
14. Centers for Disease Control and Prevention. Invasive Streptococcus pyogenes after allograft implantation, Colorado, 2003. MMWR Morb Mortal Wkly Rep 2003;52:1173–6.
15. MSNBC. Body parts snatching case sparks fears. Available at: http://www.msnbc.msn.com/id/11461578. Accessed February 21, 2006.
16. Kainer MA, Linden JV, Whaley DN, et al. Clostridium infections associated with musculoskeletal-tissue allografts. N Engl J Med 2004;350:2564–71 [Errata in N Engl J Med 2004; 351:397–8 and 351:2025].
17. Dodd RY, Notari EP 4th, Stramer SL. Current prevalence and incidence of infectious disease markers and estimated window-period risk in the American Red Cross blood donor population. Transfusion 2002;42:975–9.
18. Rigney PR. Implementation of nucleic acid testing (NAT). AATB Bulletin No. 04–42. Available at: http://www.aatb.org. September 2004. Accessed July 25, 2008.
19. Gocke DJ. Tissue donor selection and safety. Clin Orthop Relat Res 2005;435:17–21.
20. Vangsness CT Jr, Wagner PP, Moore TM, et al. Overview of safety issues concerning the preparation and processing of soft-tissue allografts. Arthroscopy 2006;22:1351–8.
21. Zou S, Dodd RY, Stramer SL, et al. Tissue Safety Study Group. Probability of viremia with HBV, HCV, HIV, and HTLV among tissue donors in the United States. N Engl J Med 2004;351:751–9.
22. Centers for Disease Control and Prevention. Update: Creutzfeldt-Jakob disease associated with cadaveric dura mater grafts – Japan, 1979–2003. MMWR Morb Mortal Wkly Rep 2003;52:1179–81.
23. Office of Inspector General. Oversight of tissue banking. January 2001. Available at: www.fda.gov/ohrms/dockets/ac/01/briefing/3736b_01.pdf. Accessed July 25, 2008.
24. US Food and Drug Administration. Guidance for industry: validation of procedures for processing of human tissues intended for transplantation. Available at: http://www.fda.gov/cber/tissue/docs.htm. March 2002. Accessed July 25, 2008.
25. US Food and Drug Administration. Tissue related documents. Available at: http://www.fda.gov/cber/tissue/docs.htm. October 30, 2006. Accessed July 25, 2008.
26. Crawford C, Kainer M, Jernigan D, et al. Investigation of postoperative allograft-associated infections in patients who underwent musculoskeletal allograft implantation. Clin Infect Dis 2005;41:195–200.

27. Veen MR, Bloem RM, Petit PL. Sensitivity and negative predictive value of swab cultures in musculoskeletal allograft procurement. Clin Orthop Relat Res 1994; 300:259–63.
28. American Association of Tissue Banks: standards for tissue banking. MacLean (VA): American Association of Tissue Banks; October, 2006.
29. Fideler BM, Vangsness CT Jr, Moore T, et al. Effects of gamma irradiation on the human immunodeficiency virus. A study in frozen human bone-patellar ligament-bone grafts obtained from infected cadavers. J Bone Joint Surg Am 1994;76: 1032–5.
30. Lemaire R, Masson JB. Risk of transmission of blood-borne viral infection in ortho-paedic and trauma surgery. J Bone Joint Surg Br 2000;82B:313–23.
31. Prolo DJ, Pedrotti PW, White DH. Ethylene oxide sterilization of bone, dura mater, and fascia lata for human transplantation. Neurosurgery 1980;6:529–39.
32. Jackson DW, Windler GE, Simon TM. Intraarticular reaction associated with the use of freeze-dried, ethylene oxide-sterilized bone-patella tendon-bone allografts in the reconstruction of the anterior cruciate ligament. Am J Sports Med 1990;18:1–11.
33. Roberts TS, Drez D Jr, McCarthy W, et al. Anterior cruciate ligament reconstruc-tion using freeze-dried, ethylene oxide-sterilized, bone-patellar tendon-bone allo-grafts. Two year results in thirty-six patients. Am J Sports Med 1991;19:35–41.
34. Steenland K, Stayner L, Greife A, et al. Mortality among workers exposed to ethylene oxide. N Engl J Med 1991;324:1402–7.
35. Smith CW, Young IS, Kearney JN. Mechanical properties of tendons: changes with sterilization and preservation. J Biomech Eng 1996;118:56–61.
36. FDA Workshop: processing of orthopedic, cardiovascular and skin allografts. Bethesda (MD), October 12, 2007. Available at: http://www.fda.gov/cber/minutes/allog101207t.htm.
37. Pruss A, Bauman B, Seibold M, et al. Validation of the sterilization procedure of allogeneic avital bone transplants using peracetic acid-ethanol. Biologicals 2001;29:59–66.
38. Pruss A, Gobel UB, Pauli G, et al. Peracetic acid-ethanol treatment of allogeneic avital bone tissue transplants—a reliable sterilization method. Ann Transplant 2003;8:34–42.
39. Scheffler SU, Scherler J, Pruss A, et al. Biomechanical comparison of human bone-patellar tendon-bone grafts after sterilization with peracetic acid ethanol. Cell Tissue Bank 2005;6:109–15.
40. Scheffler SU, Gonnermann J, Kamp J, et al. Remodeling of ACL allografts is inhibited by peracetic acid sterilization. Clin Orthop Relat Res [Epub ahead of print].
41. Campbell DG, Li P. Sterilization of HIV with irradiation: relevance to infected bone allografts. Aust N Z J Surg 1999;69:517–21.
42. Mitchell EJ, Stawarz AM, Kayacan R, et al. The effect of gamma radiation steril-ization on the fatigue crack propagation resistance of human cortical bone. J Bone Joint Surg Am 2004;86:2648–57.
43. Moroz TE, Lin EL, Summit MC, et al. Biomechanical analysis of allograft bone treated with a novel tissue sterilization process. Spine J 2006;6:34–9.
44. Nguyen H, Morgan DA, Forwood MR. Sterilization of allograft bone: is 25 kGy the gold standard for gamma irradiation? Cell Tissue Bank 2007;8:81–91.
45. Schwartz HE, Matava MJ, Proch FS, et al. The effect of gamma irradiation on an-terior cruciate ligament allograft biomechanical and biochemical properties in the caprine model at time zero and at 6 months after surgery. Am J Sports Med 2006; 34:1747–55.

46. Curran AR, Adams DJ, Gill JL, et al. The biomechanical effects of low-dose irradiation on bone-patellar tendon-bone allografts. Am J Sports Med 2004;32: 1131–5.
47. Balsly CR, Cotter AT, Williams LA, et al. Effect of low dose and moderate dose gamma irradiation on the mechanical properties of bone and soft tissue allografts. Cell Tissue Bank [Epub ahead of print].
48. Dziedzic-Goclawska A, Kaminski A, Uhrynowska-Tyszkiewicz I, et al. Irradiation as a safety procedure in tissue banking. Cell Tissue Bank 2005;6:201–19.
49. Seto A, Gatt Jr CJ, Dunn MG. Radioprotection of tendon tissue via crosslinking and free radical scavenging. Clin Orthop Relat Res [Epub ahead of print].
50. Pruss A, Keshlaf S, Smith M, et al. A novel sterilization process based on electron beam radiation does not impair the mechanical properties of soft tissue allografts. Available at: http://www.aatb.org/files/2007abstract19.pdf. Accessed July 25, 2008.
51. Akkus O, Belaney RM, Das P. Free radial scavenging alleviates the biomechanical impairment of gamma radiation sterilized bone tissue. J Orthop Res 2005; 23:838–45.
52. Hawkins CL, Davies MJ. Oxidative damage to collagen and related substrates by metal ion/hydrogen peroxide systems: random attack or site-specific damage? Biochim Biophys Acta 1997;1360:84–96.
53. Grieb TA, Forng RY, Bogdansky S, et al. High-dose gamma irradiation for soft tissue allografts: high margin of safety with biomechanical integrity. J Orthop Res 2006;24:1011–8.
54. Kattaya SA, Akkus O, Slama J. Radioprotectant and radiosensitizer effects on sterility of gamma-irradiated bone. Clin Orthop Relat Res 2008 May [Epub ahead of print].
55. Jones DB, Huddleston PM, Zobitz ME, et al. Mechanical properties of patellar tendon allografts subjected to chemical sterilization. Arthroscopy 2007;23:400–4.
56. Schimizzi A, Wedemeyer M, Odell T, et al. Effects of a novel sterilization process on soft tissue mechanical properties for anterior cruciate ligament allografts. Am J Sports Med 2007;35:612–6.
57. DePaula CA, Truncale KG, Gertzman AA, et al. Effects of hydrogen peroxide clearing procedures on bone graft osteoconductivity and mechanical properties. Cell Tissue Bank 2005;6:287–98.
58. Sterling JC, Meyers MC, Calvo RD. Allograft failure in cruciate ligament reconstruction. Follow-up evaluation of eighteen patients. Am J Sports Med 1995;23: 173–8.
59. Cornu O, Banse X, Docquier PL, et al. Effect of freeze-drying and gamma irradiation on the mechanical properties of human cancellous bone. J Orthop Res 2000;18:426–31.
60. American Academy of Orthopaedic Surgeons. Advisory Statement #1011: use of musculoskeletal tissue allografts. Available at: http://www.aaos.org/about/papers/advistmt/1011.asp. Accessed July 25, 2008.
61. Joyce MJ. Safety and FDA regulations for musculoskeletal allografts: perspective of an orthopaedic surgeon. Clin Orthop Relat Res 2005;435:22–30.

Biology of Allograft Incorporation

Michael J. Eagan, MD, David R. McAllister, MD*

KEYWORDS

• Allograft • Incorporation • Autograft • Biology • Immunology

Allograft tissues play a vital role in orthopedic surgery, and in particular, sports medicine. Their use in reconstructive knee procedures, such as anterior and posterior cruciate ligament reconstructions and posterolateral corner reconstructions, has been well documented.[1–4] For many procedures, allograft reconstruction may be offered to the patient as an alternative to autograft tissue harvesting. Allografts offer the advantage of decreased operative time (because there is no need to harvest allograft tissue) and also eliminate the complications and morbidity associated with autograft harvesting.[5] For other procedures, such as reconstruction of large osteochondral or meniscal defects, no suitable autograft options exist, and allografts are the only option.

In recent years, there has been an increase in the number of tissue donors annually and an even larger increase in the number of musculoskeletal tissues recovered. According to the American Association of Tissue Banks (AATB), there were 17,010 donors recovered from accredited tissue banks in 1996, 20,490 in 2001, and 23,295 in 2003. In the same period, distribution of musculoskeletal tissues from these donors increased from 337,338 in 1996 to 710,064 in 2001 and 1,279,000 in 2003.[6] According to a recent survey of members of the American Orthopaedic Society for Sports Medicine (AOSSM), allograft tissue is used widely among practitioners, with 86% of respondents reporting that they use allografts in their clinical practices.[7,8] It has been estimated by the AOSSM that there were approximately 60,000 allografts used in knee reconstruction procedures alone in 2005.[6]

Given the widespread acceptance and use of allograft tissues, it is critical that a thorough understanding of the basic science of allograft incorporation exist. To this end, much research has been devoted to the topic. It is important to realize that not all allograft tissues are alike, and different tissues behave uniquely in the biologic milieu of the human body. This chapter explores several common musculoskeletal allografts frequently used in sports medicine and orthopedic surgery and the biology of graft incorporation.

UCLA Department of Orthopaedic Surgery, David Geffen School of Medicine at UCLA, CHS, Box 956902, Los Angeles, CA 90095-6902, USA
* Corresponding author.
E-mail address: uclaorthopaedics@gmail.com (D.R. McAllister).

Clin Sports Med 28 (2009) 203–214
doi:10.1016/j.csm.2008.10.009
0278-5919/08/$ – see front matter. Published by Elsevier Inc.

sportsmed.theclinics.com

BONE ALLOGRAFT

Although not unique to orthopedic sports medicine, a discussion of bone allograft is warranted, given the frequency of its use in all areas of orthopedic surgery. Bone is the second most commonly transplanted tissue after blood transfusion.[9] It is estimated that there are approximately 500,000 bone grafting procedures performed annually in the United States, with approximately 200,000 of these involving allografts.[9]

The process of bone graft incorporation (**Table 1**) has been described in terms of 5 stages of healing.[10] Stage 1, or the inflammatory stage, is marked by the arrival of various inflammatory cells to the bone graft site, attracted via the common mechanism of chemotaxis. Stage 2 is marked by the differentiation of host mesenchymal cells into osteoblasts, while stage 3, or osteoinduction, involves the functioning of both osteoblasts and osteoclasts. Stage 4 is osteoconduction, in which new bone forms over an existing scaffold. Stage 5 is remodeling, and it is the final stage. This process continues for several years after graft implantation.

Bone grafts have been noted to have both osteoconductive and osteoinductive effects.[10] Osteoconductivity refers to a graft's passive ability to act as a framework onto which host bone growth may occur. Osteoinductivity, on the other hand, refers to the ability to actively stimulate host bone growth. This stimulation relies on various biologic growth factors present in living bone, including bone morphogenetic proteins (BMPs), transforming growth factor-beta (TGF-β), insulin-like growth factor (IGF), and platelet-derived growth factor (PDGF). The presence of these biologic signal molecules stimulates bone healing and formation by inducing osteoblastic differentiation of mesenchymal cells and stimulating the production of collagen, cartilage matrix, and ossified bone formation. These factors are present to different degrees in various allograft tissues and may be affected by pre-implantation handling, storage, and sterilization.[6]

The 2 most commonly used bone allografts are cancellous and cortical bone (**Table 2**). Cancellous bone is used commonly for grafting of non-unions and for filling bony defects. It has the advantage of rapid incorporation and revascularization via a process that has been described as one of creeping substitution.[11] In this mode of incorporation, host osteoblasts invade the graft and rapidly lay down new bone on top of donor trabeculae, which are subsequently resorbed and remodeled. It has been estimated that remodeling of cancellous bone graft continues for 2 to 3 years after implantation.[12–14]

Cortical bone incorporation is a much slower process, however. Cortical bone is denser than cancellous bone and is often used as structural or load-bearing bone graft. Incorporation is initiated when the osteon borders of the graft are resorbed. This causes a delayed weakening of the graft material and is a potential source of graft

Table 1	
Stages of Bone Graft Healing	
Stage	Action
1. Inflammation	Vasodilation; inflammatory cells attracted by chemotaxis
2. Osteoblast differentiation	Mesenchymal cells differentiate into osteoblasts
3. Osteoinduction	Osteoblasts and osteoclasts are stimulated to begin process of bone healing
4. Osteoconduction	Bone begins to form over scaffold of graft
5. Remodeling	Resorption and new bone formation continues for extended period of time

Table 2
Properties of Bone Allograft

Graft	Osteoconduction	Osteoinduction	Structural Integrity	Rate of Incorporation	Immunogenicity
Autograft - cancellous	Excellent	Good	Poor	Fast	None
Autograft - cortical	Fair	Fair	Excellent	Slow	None
Allograft - fresh	Good (cancellous)	Good	Poor (cancellous)	Intermediate	High
Allograft - freeze-dried	Fair	Poor	Poor (cancellous)	Intermediate	Low
Allograft- fresh-frozen	Good (cancellous)	Fair	Poor (cancellous)	Intermediate	Intermediate
DBM	Fair	Good	Poor	Rapid	Low

failure or fracture.[15,16] The existing haversian systems are remodeled by gradual resorption and deposition of new bone, which eventually restores strength to the graft. It is believed that remodeling is confined to the osteon borders only, while internal lamellae are maintained.[10] Complete incorporation and remodeling of cortical bone grafts may not occur, but the clinical significance of this is not clear.[17]

When transplanting any allograft tissue, the issue of immunogenicity must always be considered. Because of the complex nature of bone, several potential antigenic sources are available, including both cellular and extracellular matrix components.[10] The most powerful immunogenic response is generated by donor bone marrow cells in the graft. These cells are recognized as foreign by host T lymphocytes, which respond with a cell-mediated immune response. Furthermore, Type I collagen, proteoglycans, and other components of extracellular matrix stimulate both a cell-mediated and humoral immune response.[18,19] As with other transplanted tissues, the degree of immune response is related to major histocompatibility complex (MHC) markers and host compatibility.[20]

In addition to the issue of host-graft immunologic concerns, there is also a concern of disease transmission.[21–24] For these reasons, allografts are commonly treated to reduce the risk of infection, although these treatments frequently alter the structural properties of the tissues.[25–27] The most commonly used bone grafts are fresh, freeze-dried, or fresh frozen. Fresh allografts are implanted without pretreatment or sterilization. They carry the highest risk of disease transmission and the highest immunogenic potential but have the advantage of maintaining structural integrity. They also carry the highest osteoinductive potential, as they contain the most BMP and biologically active proteins.[10] Freeze-dried bone is most commonly used in the form of cancellous bone croutons. The process of freeze-drying has been shown to nearly eliminate the risk of disease transmission while also altering the antigenic properties of MHC markers.[28,29] This has the effect of significantly reducing the immunogenic potential of the tissue, but freeze-drying also structurally weakens the bone and eliminates the osteoinductive properties of the graft.[10,29] Fresh-frozen tissue is a third option. It has an intermediate immunogenicity, intermediate osteoinductive capacity, and less loss of structural integrity compared with freeze-drying. It does, however, also carry a higher risk of disease transmission than freeze-dried grafts.[10,30]

Various commercially available products have also been developed and marketed as both bone graft substitutes and bone graft extenders. One commonly used product is demineralized bone matrix (DBM). DBM is prepared by acid extraction of whole bone to remove the mineralized component, leaving behind the extracellular matrix, collagen, non-collagenous protein, BMP, TGF-β, IGF, and other growth factors.[31] It has both osteoconductive and osteoinductive properties. Other products are marketed as bone graft extenders and attempt to capitalize on the osteoinductive properties of various growth factors. Recombinant human BMP-2 (rhBMP-2) is one product commonly used as an adjunct to bone grafting in spinal fusion procedures. When it is used in conjunction with cancellous allograft, fusion rates have been shown to approach those achieved with iliac crest autograft, which is historically the gold standard.[32–36]

TENDON ALLOGRAFT

Tendon allograft is one of the most commonly used tissues in sports medicine procedures. Grafts are available from several sources, including Achilles tendon, hamstring, and patellar tendon. Although tendon grafts have been applied to a variety of surgical procedures, this discussion focuses on anterior cruciate ligament (ACL) reconstruction.

There has been a great deal of study evaluating the incorporation and remodeling of implanted tendon allograft.[37,38] These studies have involved animal models[38] or have studied grafts recovered from patients during postmortem examination or during revision surgical procedures.[37] It has been shown that implanted tendon grafts act as a Type I collagen scaffold which host tissue envelops and invades, in a process described as "ligamentization."[39–41] In the case of ACL reconstruction, invasion of the graft begins in the bone tunnels and involves revascularization as well as synovial investment of the tendon. This is followed by fibroblast and synovial cell invasion of the tissue, which serves to repopulate the tendon with host cells.[42,43] These cells then gradually remodel, incorporate, and maintain the matrix of the graft. Compared with autograft ACL reconstruction, allograft incorporation seems to proceed in a similar, but slower, manner.[37,42–44] One study that evaluated retrieved allografts found that the central portion of the graft remained essentially acellular, even after 2 years of implantation, and there was incomplete healing to the bone.[45]

As noted previously, any foreign tissue has the ability to stimulate an immunologic reaction after implantation within a host, and this is certainly the case with tendon allograft. This has been seen in studies that implanted fresh grafts with viable cells, stimulating host lymphocyte invasion, hyperemia, and graft rejection.[42] As with bone graft, this intense response is probably related to the expression of major histo-compatibility markers present on the surface of viable allograft tendon cells. For this reason, implantation of fresh tendon allografts is generally not performed. Fortunately, deep-freezing has been shown to kill graft cells and sufficiently modify the structure of their MHC markers, without altering the initial structural and mechanical properties of the graft.[46,47] Implantation of deep-frozen, nonviable grafts is, therefore, possible without significant concern of host rejection. Furthermore, one study examined the implantation of fresh, viable tendon allografts in an animal model and found that donor DNA was no longer detectable in the implanted graft after 4 weeks, suggesting that donor cells had already been replaced by those of the host.[48] This study further called into question the need to implant a viable graft.

Although implantation of deep-frozen tendon grafts does not elicit the robust immune response seen with fresh viable grafts, multiple studies have uncovered a more occult response that may be present.[49,50] One such study identified the presence of anti-donor IgG antibodies in 38% of patients implanted with deep-frozen tendon allograft, indicating a host humoral-mediated immune response.[51] There was, however, no difference in clinical outcome between this group and those that did not manifest antibodies. Other studies have also described immune responses that are localized and limited in scope after use of nonviable grafts, and it has been rarely reported that acute rejection is a cause of graft failure in ACL reconstruction.[52] This low-level response of the host immune system may, however, explain the delayed and often incomplete incorporation of tendon allograft and may ultimately be a cause of graft failure.[41]

MENISCAL ALLOGRAFT

Unlike bone and tendon grafts, no acceptable autograft option exists to replace meniscal tissue. This problem underscores the importance of allograft tissue as the only acceptable option for meniscal replacement.

Owing to the unique function of the meniscus, correct size and shape matching between patient and donor is important in achieving good outcomes. Once a correct match has been made, meniscal tissue is implanted into the host via both soft tissue attachment and, in some cases, bone attachment as well. Healing and incorporation of meniscus have been shown to occur at both the soft-tissue sites as well as via the subchondral bone plugs.[53–55] In the case of bone plugs, creeping substitution is responsible for graft incorporation. As stated previously, host osteoblasts invade the graft and line trabeculae, forming new bone while simultaneous resorption and remodeling occur. At the periphery of the graft, fibrovascular invasion occurs, which serves to anchor the meniscus to the joint capsule and surrounding soft tissues and also helps to re-establish the vascular nature of the peripheral portion of the graft.[53,54,56]

The importance of maintaining viable donor cells in the implanted graft is somewhat controversial. Theoretically, viable donor cells may maintain the extracellular matrix of the graft and lead to superior structural and mechanical properties and thus improved clinical outcomes. Following this reasoning, it was once believed that rapid implantation within 12 hours of graft harvesting was necessary to maintain viable donor cells.[57] Using basic tissue culture techniques, however, it has been shown that fresh allografts maintained in Dulbecco's Modified Eagle Medium with 20% serum preserve viable cells capable of matrix production for up to 2 weeks after harvesting.[58] This extended period of time allows for improved surgical planning, patient selection, and donor tissue testing.

Cryopreservation has also been advocated as a means of maintaining viable donor cells over an extended period of time.[53,56] Using deep-freezing techniques in the presence of cryoprotectants such as glycerol and dimethyl sulfoxide (DMSO), allografts can be maintained in tissue banks while donor screening and patient matching take place. Biomechanical studies have shown that cryopreservation does not significantly alter the structural or mechanical properties of the graft, but only 10% to 30% of cells remain viable with this process.[54,59]

As stated earlier, the importance of viable donor cells in meniscal allografts is controversial. Several studies examining recovered meniscal allografts have demonstrated that after a brief period of implantation, donor cells and DNA are either no longer detectable or are detectable in much smaller amounts than host cells and DNA.[60] For this reason, many believe that viable donor cells are not necessary for a successful clinical outcome following meniscal implantation. This has led to an increase in popularity of deep-frozen allografts, which maintain the structural and mechanical properties of fresh and cryopreserved grafts but lack viable donor cells.[53] An additional advantage of deep-frozen allografts is that donor antigen markers within the bone plugs are altered by the freezing process and are thus less immunogenic than other forms.[46] Currently, no good evidence exists to suggest a benefit with regard to clinical outcome between viable versus nonviable meniscal grafts.[58] Finally, freeze-dried (lyophilized) and sterilized meniscal allografts are not recommended because of inferior mechanical properties caused by the freeze-drying and sterilization process.[61]

The fate of implanted meniscal tissue is not entirely clear. While host cell repopulation has been shown to occur, the extent of cellularity is variable and incomplete.[54] Furthermore, repopulation of the graft is believed to occur by fibroblast invasion, and the ability of these cells to maintain the complex and important extracellular matrix of the graft is questionable. One study determined that, on average, implanted meniscal allografts show an increase in water content of approximately 25%, with greater than 50% decrease in proteoglycan content.[56] Presumably, this altered biochemical profile should adversely affect graft survivability, but this has not been proven clinically. Other studies have shown incomplete incorporation of meniscal grafts, graft extrusion, and even meniscal shrinkage.[62]

Although the cancellous bone plugs associated with meniscal allografts can trigger a robust host immune response similar to other forms of bone graft, it is often stated that the meniscal tissue itself is "immunoprivileged." This is presumed to be related to a low cell number within a dense environment of extracellular matrix, essentially iso-lating the cells from the host's immune system.[53] Several studies have challenged this belief, however. One such experiment examined meniscal biopsy specimens obtained following graft implantation.[62] It showed that low numbers of host lymphocytes had invaded the graft and surrounding tissues, indicating a mild immune response. Furthermore, there have been case reports of infrequent frank rejection of meniscal allografts, although this appears to be rare.[12] From the available data, it appears that a subtle local immune response is common, but the clinical significance of this is not known.[62] Some researchers have suggested that this could be the cause of altered biochemical graft composition and could ultimately affect graft incorporation, remodeling, and longevity.[41]

OSTEOCHONDRAL ALLOGRAFTS

Osteochondral allografts are primarily used to repair large defects in the articular surface of the knee related to trauma or osteochondritis dissecans (OCD). It is typically considered a salvage procedure for lesions that are too large to be amenable to other modes of treatment[63,64] or in cases where other treatments have failed. Lesions treated by osteochondral allografting are usually large (>4 cm^2), unifocal, and traumatic in nature, rather than degenerative.[63] The typical patient is young (20–30 years) and active, with a large traumatic or OCD lesion involving the medial femoral condyle.

The structure of osteochondral allograft comprises a bony component and a cartilaginous articular component. The subchondral cancellous bone supports the important articular component and is critical for incorporation into the host bone.[10]

Osteochondral grafts are size-matched by the tissue bank and implanted after an appropriately sized graft becomes available. They are typically trimmed to size and implanted into prepared regions of subchondral bone that have been prepared and sized to match the donor graft. They can be fixed in place with bioabsorbable screws or anchors, although commercially available instrument sets rely primarily on press-fit fixation and do not necessarily require fixation implants. Incorporation of the subchondral portion of osteochondral allografts is similar for other forms of bone graft.[11] Donor bone acts as an osteoconductive scaffold, onto which host osteoblasts invade and remodel the bone. This creeping substitution probably continues for several years after implantation.[12,14]

In contrast to the subchondral portion of the graft, remodeling and incorporation of the articular component of an osteochondral graft would be detrimental to its function. Specifically, host invasion of articular cartilage would presumably replace hyaline cartilage with inferior fibrocartilage, and graft failure would be inevitable. Several studies have demonstrated superior clinical outcomes when viable donor cells are present during implantation.[8,65] Presumably, the ability of donor cells to maintain the extracellular matrix of articular cartilage is critical to preventing host invasion and remodeling of the graft. An important animal study revealed that 1 year after implantation of an osteochondral allograft, those grafts that maintained higher numbers of donor cells had superior structural properties.[66] The importance of chondrocyte viability to graft survival is supported by evidence that fresh osteochondral allografts have superior structural properties when compared with frozen grafts.[61] Furthermore, storage time has a negative effect on cell viability. One study determined that percent cell viability decreases from 100% at day 1 following harvest to 98% at day 8 to 80% at day 15 to 64% at day 45 and 52% at day 60.[61] Clearly, implantation of fresh allografts is necessary to maximize viable chondrocytes, and chondrocyte viability can be increased by decreasing the storage time of these grafts.

To maximize viable donor cells, many researchers have advocated implantation of fresh allograft immediately after tissue harvesting.[12] Certainly, the need to maintain viable cells precludes any sterilization from occurring, so these grafts offer the very real risk of communicable disease transmission. Others have advocated cryopreservation of grafts using glycerol and DMSO; however, results have been rather disappointing, with most studies finding less than 50% cell viability after thawing.[67,68] Other investigators have demonstrated up to 70% cell viability after 28 days when allografts are refrigerated in culture media.[69] Furthermore, this method of storage does not seem to adversely affect biochemical composition or structural properties of the graft.[69]

The need to maintain viable cell populations in osteochondral allografts leads to many challenges. As stated earlier, it is not possible to sterilize these grafts, which increases the risk of disease transmission. To lessen the risk of communicable disease, it is necessary to screen and culture donor tissue prior to implantation. In general, these grafts are released from tissue banks after approximately 14 days, assuming final screening tests and cultures are negative. Once cleared for release, it is necessary to rapidly implant the grafts to maximize viable donor cells. This process is further complicated by the need to size-match patients and grafts, which necessitates that a recipient list be maintained.

Although it is generally agreed that viable grafts are superior to nonviable grafts, the long-term fate of donor cells is not entirely clear. Grafts have been evaluated by biopsy at several time points, and cell viability has been shown to decrease with time. In one study of fresh osteochondral allografts, cell viability decreased from 96% at 12 months to 37% at 6 years,[65] although the clinical significance of this decline is not known. Another study has demonstrated that load bearing of an osteochondral graft has positive effects on cell viability,[70] which may indicate that grafts placed in weight-bearing regions will fare better than those in other locations.

Similar to the discussion of meniscal allografts, it is commonly believed that articular cartilage is immunoprivileged. This is believed to be related to the large ratio of extracellular matrix to donor cells. Because the majority of donor chondrocytes are embedded deep within the matrix, they are never exposed to host immunity. As with meniscal tissue, however, evidence exists that a limited host immune response may occur in a majority of patients, but the clinical significance of this is not known.[71] The major source of immune response with osteochondral grafts, though, is the subchondral bone.[72] As discussed earlier, bone contains many potential antigens, and the inability to freeze-dry the graft means that there is a higher propensity to develop an immune response. The most significant antigenic source is the marrow components of the subchondral bone, however, and this can be diminished by thoroughly removing all blood and marrow components from the graft by pulse lavage.[41] When this is performed, the host's immune response to subchondral bone appears to be localized and self-limited and rarely leads to graft rejection or failure.[73]

SUMMARY

The use of allograft tissues in orthopedic sports medicine has increased dramatically in recent years. With tissue banks and safety guidelines, allograft tissue implantation has emerged as a safe and effective alternative to autograft procedures. In many instances, no acceptable autograft alternatives exist, and allograft tissue implantation is the only option available.

The successful incorporation of any allograft depends on several factors that must be identified and understood by the surgeon. These include proper patient selection, proper operative technique, and an understanding of the immunology and biology of allograft incorporation. Furthermore, it is necessary for the surgeon to be familiar with the techniques used by his or her tissue bank to store, preserve, and sterilize these allografts, and how these processes affect the viability, immunology, and structural properties of these tissues. As the number of donors and tissue transplantations continues to rise, safe and effective use of these allografts requires a thorough understanding of these key elements.

REFERENCES

1. Harner C, Olson E, Irrgang J, et al. Allograft versus autograft anterior cruciate ligament reconstruction: 3- to 5-year outcome. Clin Orthop 1996;324:134–44.
2. Nemzek J, Swenson C, Arnoczky S. Retroviral transmission by the transplantation of connective tissue allografts: An experimental study. J Bone Joint Surg Am 1994;76:1036–41.
3. Saddemi S, Frogameni A, Fenton P, et al. Comparison of perioperative morbidity of anterior cruciate ligament autografts versus allografts. Arthroscopy 1993;9:519–24.
4. Shelton W, Treacy S, Dukes A, et al. Use of allografts in knee reconstruction: I. Basic science aspects and current status. J Am Acad Orthop Surg 1998;6:165–8.
5. Kohn D. Autograft meniscus replacement: Experimental and clinical results. Knee Surg Sports Traumatol Arthrosc 1993;1:123–5.
6. McAllister D, Joyce M, Mann B. The current status of tissue regulation, procurement, processing, and sterilization. Am J Sports Med 2007;35(12):2148–58.
7. Leever Research Services. 2006 AOSSM Orthopaedic Surgical Procedure Survey on Allografts. Naperville (IL): Leever Research Services; 2006.
8. AAOS. American Academy of Orthopaedic Surgeons Advisory Statement #1011: Use of musculoskeletal tissue allografts. Available at: http://www.aaos.org/about/papers/advistmt/1011.asp. Accessed June 15, 2008.
9. Melvin J. Bone grafts and bone graft substitutes. Available at: http://www.orthopaedia.com/display/Main/Bone+grafts+and+bone+graft+substitutes. Accessed June 15, 2008.
10. Brinker M, O'Connor D. Basic Sciences. In: Miller M, editor. Review of Orthopaedics. 4th edition. Philadelphia: WB Saunders; 2004. p. 1–66.
11. Burchardt H. The biology of bone graft repair. Clin Orthop Relat Res 1983;174:28–42.
12. Backstein D, Safir O, Gross A. Allograft osteochondral transplantation: bulk graft. In: Scott N, editor. Insall & Scott: Surgery of the Knee. 4th edition. Philadelphia: Churchill Livingston-Elsevier; 2006. p. 420–32.
13. Enneking W, Campanacci D. Retrieved human allografts: A clinicopathological study. J Bone Joint Surg 2001;83A:971–86.
14. Enneking W, Mindell E. Observations on massive retrieved human allografts. J Bone Joint Surg 1991;73A:1123–42.
15. Johnson A, Eurell J, Scaeffer D. Evaluation of canine cortical bone graft remodeling. Vet Surg 2008;21(4):293–8.
16. Burchardt H, Jones H, Glowczewskie F, et al. Freeze-dried allogenic segmental cortical bone grafts in dogs. J Bone Joint Surg 1978;60:1082–90.
17. DeLuca L, Raszewski R, Tresser N, et al. The fate of preserved autogenous bone graft. Plast Reconstr Surg 1997;99(5):1324–8.
18. Elves M, Ford C. A study of the humoral immune response to massive osteochondral allografts in sheep. Clin Exp Immunol 1976;23(2):360–6.

19. Musculo D, Kawai S, Ray R. Cellular and humoral immune response analysis of bone allografted rats. J Bone Joint Surg 1976;58:826–32.
20. Reikeras D, Shegarfi H, Naper C, et al. Impact of MHC mismatch and freezing on bone graft incorporation: an experimental study in rats. J Orthop Res 2008;26(7):925–31.
21. Archibald L, Jernigan D, Kainer M. Update: Allograft-associated bacterial infections—United States. MMWB Morb Mortal Wkly Rep 2002;51:207–10.
22. Campbell D, Li P. Sterilization of HIV with irradiation: relevance to infected bone allografts. Aust N Z J Surg 1999;69:517–21.
23. Centers for Disease Control and Prevention. Invasive Streptococcus pyogenes after allograft implantation—Colorado, 2003. MMWR Morb Mortal Wkly Rep 2003;52:1173–6.
24. Centers for Disease Control and Prevention. Semiannual Report of the National Nosocomial Infection Surveillance (NNIS) System. Atlanta (GA): Centers for Disease Control and Prevention, US Dept of Health and Human Services. December 2000:11–13.
25. Brockbank K, Carpenter J, Dawson P. Effects of storage temperature on viable bioprosthetic heart valves. Cryobiology 1992;29:537–42.
26. Buck B, Malinin T. Human bone and tissue allografts. Preparation and safety. Clin Orthop 1994;303:8–17.
27. Fideler B, Vangsness C, Moore T, et al. Effects of gamma irradiation on the human immunodeficiency virus. A study in frozen human bone-patellar ligament-bone grafts obtained from infected cadavers. J Bone Joint Surg 1994;76:1032–5.
28. Graham W, Smith D, McGuire M. The use of frozen stored tendons for grafting: an experimental study. J Bone Joint Surg 1955;37A:624.
29. Greenwald A, Boden S, Goldberg V, et al. Bone graft substitutes: Facts, fiction, and applications. J Bone Joint Surg 2001;83(Suppl 2):98–103.
30. Buck B, Malinin T, Brown M. Bone Transplantation and human immunodeficiency virus. Clin Orthop 1994;303:8–17.
31. Benzel E, Leon S. Orthopaedics Surgical Management – Enhancing Cervical Spine Fusion. Surgical Module – Medscape Orthopaedics Surgical Management. Available at: http://www.medscape.com/viewprogram/161. Accessed June 15, 2008.
32. Burkus J, Hein S, Gormet M, et al. Is INFUSE bone graft substitute superior to autograft bone? An integrated analysis of clinical trials using the LT-CAGE lumbar tapered fusion device. J Spinal Disord Tech 2003;16(2):113–22.
33. Mokey B, Sandhu H. Use of recombinant human bone morphogenetic protein-2 in spinal fusion applications. Spine 2002;27(suppl):66–85.
34. Schimandle J, Boden S, Hutton W. Experimental spinal fusion with recombinant human bone morphogenetic protein-2. Spine 1995;20:1326–37.
35. David S, Gruber H, Meyer R, et al. Lumbar Spinal Fusion using recombinant human bone morphogenetic protein in the canine: A comparison of three dosages and two carriers. Spine 1999;24:1973–9.
36. Sandhu H, Toth J, Diwan A, et al. Histologic evaluation of the efficacy of rhBMP-2 compared with autograft bone in sheep spinal anterior interbody fusion. Spine 2002;27:567–75.
37. Jackson D, Corsetti J, Simon T. Biologic incorporation of allograft anterior cruciate ligament replacements. Clin Orthop Relat Res 1996;324:126–33.
38. Fromm B, Schafer B, Parsch D, et al. Reconstruction of the anterior cruciate ligament with a cryopreserved ACL allograft: A microangiographic and immuno-histochemical study in rabbits. Int Orthop 1996;20:378–82.

39. Amiel D, Kleiner J, Roux R, et al. The phenomenon of "ligamentization": anterior cruciate ligament reconstruction with autogenous patellar tendon. J Orthop Res 1986;4:162–72.
40. Arnoczky S, Tarvin G, Marshal J. Anterior cruciate ligament replacement using patellar tendon: An evaluation of graft revascularization in the dog. J Bone Joint Surg 1982;64:217–24.
41. Arnoczky S. The biology of allograft incorporation. J Knee Surg 2006;19(3): 207–14.
42. Arnoczky S, Warreb R, Ashlock M. Replacement of the anterior cruciate ligament using a patellar tendon allograft. An experimental study. J Bone Joint Surg 1986; 68A:376.
43. Drez DJ, DeLee J, Holden JP, et al. Anterior cruciate ligament reconstruction using bone-patellar tendon-bone allografts. A biological and mechanical evaluation in goats. Am J Sports Med 1991;19:256.
44. Jackson D, Grood E, Arnoczky S, et al. Freeze-dried anterior cruciate ligament allografts: Preliminary studies in a goat model. Am J Sports Med 1987;15:295.
45. Malinin T, Levitt R, Bashore C, et al. A study of retrieved allografts used to replace anterior cruciate ligaments. Arthroscopy 2002;18:163–70.
46. Friedlaender G, Strong D, Sell K. Studies on the antigenicity of bone. I. Freeze-dried and deep-frozen allografts in rabbits. J Bone Joint Surg 1976;58A:854–8.
47. Friedlaender G, Strong D, Sell K. Studies on the antigenicity of bone. II. Donor specific anti-HLA antibodies in human recipients of freeze dried allografts. J Bone Joint Surg 1984;66A:107–12.
48. Jackson D, Simon T. Donor cell survival and repopulation after intraarticular transplantation of tendon and ligament allografts. Microsc Res Tech 2002;58: 25–33.
49. Vasseur P, Rodrigo J, Stevenson S, et al. Replacement of the anterior cruciate ligament with a bone-ligament-bone anterior cruciate ligament allograft in dogs. Clin Orthop Relat Res 1987;219:268–77.
50. Jackson D, Windler G, Simon T. Intraarticular reaction associated with the use of freeze-dried, ethylene oxide-sterilized bone-patellar tendon-bone allografts in the reconstruction of the anterior cruciate ligament. Am J Sports Med 1990;18:1.
51. Schulte K, Thompson W, Jamison J, et al. The immune response to allograft anterior cruciate ligament reconstruction: Clinical correlation. Presented at AAOS Annual Meeting 1996.
52. Thompson W, Schulte K, Jamison J. Immunologic response to allograft anterior cruciate ligament reconstruction: Part I: Humoral and cellular parameters. Presented at AAOS Annual Meeting 1996.
53. Arnoczky S, DiCarlo E, O'Brien S, et al. Cellular population of deep-frozen meniscal autografts: an experimental study in the dog. Arthroscopy 1992;8:428–36.
54. Arnoczky S, McDevitt C, Schmidt M, et al. The effect of cryopreservation on canine menisci: a biochemical, morphologic, and biomechanical evaluation. J Orthop Res 1998;6:1–12.
55. Arnoczky S, Waren R, McDevitt C. Meniscal replacement using a cryopreserved allograft. An experimental study in the dog. Clin Orthop Relat Res 1990;252: 121–8.
56. Jackson D, McDevitt C, Simon T, et al. Meniscal transplantation using fresh and cryopreserved allografts. An experimental study in goats. Am J Sports Med 1992; 20:644–56.
57. Garrett J. Meniscal transplantation: A review of 43 cases with 2 to 7 year follow-up. Sports Med Arthrosc Rev 1993;1:164–7.

58. Verdonk P, Demurie A, Almquist K, et al. Transplantation of Viable Meniscal Allograft. J Bone Joint Surg 2005;87A:715–24.
59. Verdonk R, Kohn D. Harvest and conservation of meniscal allografts. Scand J Med Sci Sports 1999;9:158–9.
60. Jackson D, Whelan J, Simon T. Cell survival after transplantation of fresh meniscal allografts: DNA probe analysis in a goat model. Am J Sports Med 1993;21: 540–50.
61. Williams R, Dreesae J, Chen C. Chondrocyte survival and material properties of hypothermically stored cartilage. Am J Sports Med 2004;32:132–9.
62. Rodeo S, Seneviratne A, Suzuki K, et al. Histological analysis of human meniscal allografts: A preliminary report. J Bone Joint Surg 2000;82A:1071–82.
63. Johnson D. All about allografts. Med Gen Med 2004;6(4):23.
64. Hamlet W, Liu S, Tang R. Destruction of a cryopreserved meniscal allograft: a case for acute rejection. Arthroscopy 1997;13:517–21.
65. Czitrom A, Keating S, Gross A. The viability of articular cartilage in fresh osteo-chondral allografts after clinical transplantation. J Bone Joint Surg 1990;72A: 574–81.
66. Jackson D, Halbrecht J, Proctor C, et al. Assessment of donor cell and matrix survival in fresh articular cartilage allografts in a goat model. J Orthop Res 1996;14:255–64.
67. Malinin T, Wagner P, Lo H. Hypothermic storage and cryopreservation of carti-lage: an experimental study. Clin Orthop 1985;197:15–26.
68. Schachar N, McAllister D, Stevenson M, et al. Metabolic and biochemical status of articular cartilage following cryopreservation and transplantation: a rabbit model. J Orthop Res 1992;10:603–9.
69. Williams S, Amiel D, Ball S, et al. Prolonged storage effects in the articular carti-lage of fresh human osteochondral allografts. J Bone Joint Surg Am 2003;85: 2111–20.
70. Gole M, Poulsen D, Marzo J, et al. Chondrocyte viability in press-fit cryopre-served osteochondral allografts. J Orthop Res 2004;22:781–7.
71. Phipatanakul W, VandeVord P, Teige R, et al. Immune response in patients receiving fresh osteochondral allografts. Am J Orthop 2004;33:345–8.
72. Jackson D, Simon T, Kurzweil P, et al. Survival of cells after intra-articular trans-plantation of fresh allografts of the patellar and anterior cruciate ligaments: DNA probe analysis in a goat model. J Bone Joint Surg Am 1992;74:112–8.
73. Langer F, Czitrom A, Pritzker K, et al. The immunogenicity of fresh and frozen allogeneic bone. J Bone Joint Surg 1975;57A:216–20.

What Do We Really Know About Allografts?

Annunziato Amendola, MD[a,b,*], Mary P. Stolley, RN BSN[a]

KEYWORDS

• Allografts • Ligament • Reconstruction
• Osteochondral • Meniscal

The use of allografts in sports medicine is becoming increasingly popular, and, therefore, this issue of *Clinics in Sports Medicine* is dedicated, in a timely fashion, to the use of allografts in sports medicine. The majority of indications are related to the use of soft tissue grafts for ligament reconstruction, OC allografts for articular surface reconstruction, and meniscal allografts for meniscal transplantation. There is an increasing amount of science and literature dealing with healing and outcomes, but many questions still remain. There are a number of issues, controversies, and lack of long-term outcomes to make definitive statements on what is really known about allograft use in sports medicine.

There are number of important factors that one must consider when deciding to use allografts for soft tissue reconstruction. The risk of disease transmission and the safety of use of allograft tissue, the processing and preparation of allograft tissue, which may effect biologic and biomechanical properties, and the biologic healing and incorporation of allograft tissue once it is used in surgery are all significant concerns and considerations. These issues, as well as the use of allograft tissue within the various specific indications, are covered in detail in other sections. The purpose of this article is to look at, in a concise fashion, what is known about autograft versus allograft tissue in terms of advantages and disadvantages, morbidity, the actual biology of these 2 tissue graft types, and evidence with respect to clinical outcomes.

AUTOGRAFT VERSUS ALLOGRAFT FOR LIGAMENT RECONSTRUCTION

Allografts have been commonly used for multiple-ligament injuries to the knee because of the pure practicality and lack of autograft tissue to reconstruct the severely

---

[a] Department of Orthopaedic Surgery, University of Iowa Health Care, 200 Hawkins Dr. 01018JPP, Iowa City, IA 52242, USA
[b] University of Iowa Sports Medicine, University of Iowa Health Care, 200 Hawkins Drive, 01018JPP, Iowa City, IA 52242, USA
* Corresponding author. Department of Orthopaedic Surgery, University of Iowa Health Care, 200 Hawkins Drive, 01018JPP, Iowa City, IA 52242, USA.
E-mail address: ned-amendola@uiowa.edu (A. Amendola).

Clin Sports Med 28 (2009) 215–222
doi:10.1016/j.csm.2008.10.002
0278-5919/08/$ – see front matter © 2009 Elsevier Inc. All rights reserved.

compromised knee. Using multiple autografts in these situations would compromise the knee joint even further. Allografts have also been used in the reconstruction of the posterior cruciate ligament most commonly, again, to have enough available graft tissue for reconstruction and to produce a biomechanically stable construct for the posterior cruciate ligament. The anterior cruciate ligament (ACL) has become increasingly popular in indications in which allografts have been used, in particular for revision surgery. However, controversy exists in using allografts for primary anterior cruciate ligament reconstruction (ACLR), particularly in the young athlete. A number of issues, concerns, and questions remain in the use of allografts for ACLR.

ACL Reconstruction

Surgeons are still searching for the ideal ACLR in the athlete. Every aspect of ACLR has been studied and written on, and it is probably one of the most popular subjects with respect to the number of publications in the literature. The type of graft, allograft versus autograft, remains a significant area of interest and research with respect to ACLR. The search continues for the ideal graft substitute that will reproduce the biologic and biomechanical characteristics of the normal ACL. Some of these ideal qualities would include the ability to heal and incorporate into the host tissues and revascularize, allowing the patient's return to sport participation quickly; low surgical-site morbidity, risk of infection , and disease transmission; appropriate size and length for reconstruction; and ready availability for the number of surgical procedures that are performed.

Currently, the autografts that are used most commonly include the patellar tendon graft, the hamstrings (gracilis and semitendinosis) graft, and, much less frequently, the quadriceps tendon graft. In terms of allografts, the most common grafts that are used include bone-patellar tendon-bone constructs, Achilles tendon grafts, and soft tissue grafts that can be derived from hamstring, tibialis anterior or posterior, and peroneal tendons.

DONOR-SITE MORBIDITY

Numerous clinical studies have shown relatively good long-term results using bone-tendon-bone (BTB) autografts and hamstring autografts.[1] Despite the clinical success in using autografts, both BTB and hamstring autografts are associated with a significant amount of donor-site morbidity. These include anterior knee pain, which is common in both procedures, and kneeling pain. Spindler and colleagues[1] did a systematic review of the literature, which demonstrated that there was a similar incidence of anterior knee pain using patellar tendon and hamstring autograft and a more significant incidence of kneeling pain using patellar tendon autograft. In addition, anterior and anterolateral numbness when an anterior incision is used, because of injury to the pre-patellar branch of the saphenous nerve, causes consistent skin abnormalities in these patients. Additional complications have been reported with the patellar tendon harvest, which can be quite severe, including a patellar tendon fracture[2,3] and infrapatellar fibrosis.[4–6] One of the main issues with hamstring autograft is harvesting of the hamstring tendon itself. Some investigators have gone to a more proximal and posterior approach to the hamstring tendon because of concern about the difficulty of harvest.[7] Because of the gastrocnemius attachments of the hamstring tendons, particularly the semitendinosis, there is a risk of rupture of the tendon when trying to harvest the tendon in a closed fashion. This obviously yields a very short graft that is not useable for ACLR.

These issues do not exist with allografts in terms of difficulty with graft harvest, skin denervation, and increased sensitivity from the harvest site, risk to the extensor mechanism, and inadequate amount of tissue, as presented earlier.

BIOLOGIC INCORPORATION

It is important for the orthopedic surgeon to understand the differences in the biomechanical and biologic properties of autografts and allografts during healing. Incorporation of a bone-tendon construct or soft tissue graft is essential for long-term success of ACLR. Several studies have examined the process by which an allograft heals after ACLR.[8–11] During graft healing and incorporation into bone, allograft revascularization and maturation have been shown to be slower than those in autografts.[10] In a study by Jackson and colleagues in goats, it was demonstrated that the structural and material properties of autografts and allografts at time zero were similar but were different after implantation at 6 months. The allografts demonstrated a greater decrease in their implantation structural properties, a slower rate of biologic incorporation, and prolonged presence of an inflammatory response. In contrast, autografts demonstrate a more robust biologic response, improved stability, and increased strength-to-failure values. Delayed biologic incorporation seems to be a common theme in the literature.[12,13] In a study comparing magnetic resonance imaging (MRI) between autografts and allografts at 12 and 24 months, a decreased rate of vascularization of the allogeneic tendons was shown.[14] Malinin suggested that it may take up to 3 years for complete maturation of the allograft based on retrieved grafts; Nikolaou also showed that the autografts lagged behind in failure strength up to 24 weeks in an animal model but were similar to autografts by 36 weeks.[12,13] Allografts that require bone-to-bone healing are also slower and weaker with incorporation because they first undergo osteonecrosis of the bone plug followed by incorporation of the graft, shown by radiographic and histologic analysis of the tibial tunnel after allograft ACLR in goats.[15] In a recent study in sheep ACL, Scheffler and colleagues[16] determined in a tendon-bone healing model (soft tissue grafts) that allograft remodeling was delayed in ACLR and resulted in reduced long-term stability and mechanical function compared with autograft ACLR and recommended using caution with early aggressive rehabilitation. Therefore, in summary, the healing and mechanical properties of allografts are inferior to those of autografts for tendon-bone healing and for ACLR in vitro. This should raise some clinical concerns when extrapolating this information to performing ACLR in the athlete with aggressive rehabilitation and early return to sports.

CLINICAL OUTCOMES

Despite the physiologic and mechanical inferiority of allografts in vitro, many studies have shown no difference clinically in the stability and functionality of the different grafts.[17–22] There are concerns with some of these studies, although some are prospective randomized control trials (RCTs). With respect to ACLR, there are many potential advantages in using allograft tissue, as noted in **Tables 1** and **2**. The most significant consideration to take into account with allograft use is the clinical outcome, which includes achieving stability and optimal results that are at least comparable to those using autograft tissue. There should obviously be a significant advantage in using allograft to overcome any significant disadvantages. In a recent meta-analysis of the clinical literature on ACLR using allografts, the authors had some overall concerns with the use of allograft tissue for primary ACLR.[23] They concluded that the clinical results for stability were significantly poorer for all allografts, BTB, or soft tissue allografts. The failure rate (>5 mm laxity) was 2 to 3 times greater for allografts than autografts.

One of the main questions for primary ACLR allograft comes in its use in the young athlete, who is usually rehabilitated very aggressively and returns to play very early because function is regained quickly.

Table 1
Summary of advantages and disadvantages of allograft ACL reconstruction
Advantages
No donor-site morbidity
Variable grafts (ability to choose bone-tendon construct vs. soft tissue alone)
Decreased surgical morbidity (time, incisions)
Decreased postoperative pain and improved rehabilitation
Disadvantages
Possible risk of infection and disease transmission
Immunologic response to the allograft
Delayed healing and graft incorporation
Increased cost

There appears to be an increasing number of studies involving case series as of 2008, indicating a higher failure rate in this group of athletes. In addition, Kaeding and colleagues[24] from the MOON (Multicenter Orthopedic Outcomes Network) presented a regression analysis of cases from one surgeon and compared outcomes in autografts versus allografts. The ACLR were performed with soft tissue grafts, and the authors concluded that younger, more active patients undergoing allograft ACLR had a significantly higher risk of graft failure (**Fig. 1**).

OSTEOCHONDRAL ALLOGRAFT RESURFACING

Focal articular cartilage loss in the knee in young, active patients can be a significant, debilitating condition that is difficult to treat. These patients are generally very active, with significant demands for activity and routine activities of daily living. As a result, arthroplasty is not a good option. Although several non-arthroplasty options are available, in cases in which bone loss is present and a large amount of articular surface is involved, OC allografts are an ideal option. Realignment is always to be considered if there is compartmental overload. OC allograft transplantation has become an important and viable treatment alternative for full-thickness OC defects. A number of studies have supported its clinical efficacy, particularly for OC defects greater than 3 cm in

Table 2
Summary of advantages and disadvantages of autograft ACL reconstruction
Advantages
Improved biologic healing and incorporation
Improved outcomes with decreased laxity
Decreased cost
Improved ability to return to pre-injury sport level
Disadvantages
Donor-site morbidity
Increased surgical morbidity and complications of graft harvest
Increased postoperative anterior knee pain
Decreased rehabilitation

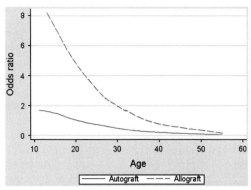

Fig. 1. Odds ratio for autograft versus allograft by age for the combined MOON cohort. (*From* Kaeding CC, Pedroza A, Aros BC, et al. Independent predictors of ACL reconstruction failure from the MOON prospective longitudinal cohort. Presented at the American Orthopaedic Society for Sports Medicine. Orlando, Florida, July 10–13, 2008; with permission.)

diameter and 1 cm in depth.[25–30] Allograft tissue can come in various shapes and sizes and can reproduce a custom articular surface for the patient, be it the knee, ankle, or other joints. Fresh OC transplantation was popularized by Alan Gross, who has reported good to excellent results for follow-up (FU) greater than 20 years.[31,32] Gross popularized fresh OC transplantation in an attempt to maintain viable chondrocytes that could maintain the cartilage matrix of the allograft cartilage.

Fresh-frozen specimens have typically been used for massive osseous defects that require large allograft specimens; such specimens contain no viable bone or cartilage cells.[33] Fresh-preserved allografts have become popular since 1998, mainly because investigators felt there was a window of time in which the chondrocytes could remain viable (up to 30 days post-retrieval). Chondrocyte viability at the time of implantation continues to be in question[34] but does not seem to be related to clinical outcomes. In recent clinical follow-ups of case series, there seems to be reasonable clinical success after early follow-up, with up to 84% good or excellent outcomes. In these cases, the implantation occurred between 14 and 42 days. It remains to be seen whether the long-term success in these cases matches the results of fresh transplantation reported by Gross and colleagues.[35–37]

The long-term durability of osteoarticular autografts or allografts is thought to depend on the function of cartilage extracellular matrix synthesis by the chondrocytes that survive the transplantation and surgical procedure.[38–41] In a 2008 article[36] with explants at various times from 1 to 25 years after fresh OC transplantation, Gross and colleagues found that the early failures had nonviable chondrocytes and lack of bony incorporation. In the late failures (up to 25 years), they found viable chondrocytes and allograft bone that had been taken over by the host bone. Storage conditions are considered critical for maintaining chondrocyte viability. Freezing cartilage sharply decreases chondrocyte viability and may disrupt the extracellular matrix.[38,42–44] In contrast, storage at 4°C does no significant harm to the matrix and is thought to better preserve chondrocyte viability. Results from several studies indicate that the majority of chondrocytes remain viable for 14 to 60 days in cartilage stored in serum-free culture medium at 4°C.[38,41,44,45] However, more recent studies have questioned the actual viability and ability of the viable chondrocytes to produce a matrix after retrieval and before implantation.[34,46] There seems to be both in vitro and in vivo support for the fact that reimplantation as soon as possible after retrieval optimizes chondrocyte viability and function.

MENISCAL ALLOGRAFTS

Meniscus transplantation is accepted as a treatment for the symptomatic, meniscus-deficient knee. There seems to be a significant amount of supportive research that joint function may be improved by the procedure in medium- to long-term (ie, 10-year) follow-up. Many areas are still under investigation, including optimal sizing and long-term impact on the progression of arthritic change. Meniscal transplantation has become increasingly more popular and successful in terms of reported outcomes over the recent past.[47] Verdonk and colleagues[48] in their survivorship analysis reported on 100 procedures in 96 patients; results showed that pain relief and functional improvement persist in approximately 70% of patients at 10-year follow-up. Osteotomy to unload the meniscus also showed a protective effect. Overall, the literature describes good or excellent results in approximately 85% of meniscal allograft transplantations.[49] Results are generally better in the knee with ACL stability, good alignment, and less arthrosis (early post-meniscectomy). Medial versus lateral meniscus transplantation shows similar outcomes.

Based largely on clinical series, meniscal allograft transplantation appears to relieve pain and improve joint function in the majority of patients. Longer-term follow-up is required to determine the optimum surgical technique, timing of transplantation, and effect on progression of arthrosis.

REFERENCES

1. Spindler KP, Kuhn JE, Freedman KB, et al. Anterior cruciate ligament reconstruction autograft choice: bone-tendon-bone versus hamstring: does it really matter? A systematic review. Am J Sports Med 2004;32(8):1986–95.
2. Lee GH, McCulloch P, Cole BJ, et al. The incidence of acute patellar tendon harvest complications for anterior cruciate ligament reconstruction. Arthroscopy 2008;24(2):162–6.
3. Marumoto JM, Mitsunaga MM, Richardson AB, et al. Late patellar tendon ruptures after removal of the central third for anterior cruciate ligament reconstruction. A report of two cases. Am J Sports Med 1996;24(5):698–701.
4. Atkinson TS, Atkinson PJ, Mendenhall HV, et al. Patellar tendon and infrapatellar fat pad healing after harvest of an ACL graft. J Surg Res 1998;79(1):25–30.
5. Tang G, Niitsu M, Ikeda K, et al. Fibrous scar in the infrapatellar fat pad after arthroscopy: MR imaging. Radiat Med 2000;18(1):1–5.
6. Unterhauser FN, Bosch U, Zeichen J, et al. Alpha-smooth muscle actin containing contractile fibroblastic cells in human knee arthrofibrosis tissue. Winner of the AGA-DonJoy Award 2003. Arch Orthop Trauma Surg 2004;124(9):585–91.
7. Prodromos CC, Fu FH, Howell SM, et al. Controversies in soft-tissue anterior cruciate ligament reconstruction: grafts, bundles, tunnels, fixation, and harvest. J Am Acad Orthop Surg 2008;16(7):376–84.
8. Arnoczky SP, Warren RF, Ashlock MA. Replacement of the anterior cruciate ligament using a patellar tendon allograft. An experimental study. J Bone Joint Surg Am 1986;68(3):376–85.
9. Jackson DW, Corsetti J, Simon TM. Biologic incorporation of allograft anterior cruciate ligament replacements. Clin Orthop Relat Res 1996;324:126–33.
10. Jackson DW, Grood ES, Goldstein JD, et al. A comparison of patellar tendon autograft and allograft used for anterior cruciate ligament reconstruction in the goat model. Am J Sports Med 1993;21(2):176–85.

11. Zhang CL, Fan HB, Xu H, et al. Histological comparison of fate of ligamentous insertion after reconstruction of anterior cruciate ligament: autograft vs. allograft. Chin J Traumatol 2006;9(2):72–6.
12. Malinin TI, Levitt RL, Bashore C, et al. A study of retrieved allografts used to replace anterior cruciate ligaments. Arthroscopy 2002;18(2):163–70.
13. Nikolaou PK, Seaber AV, Glisson RR, et al. Anterior cruciate ligament allograft transplantation. Long-term function, histology, revascularization, and operative technique. Am J Sports Med 1986;14(5):348–60.
14. Muramatsu K, Hachiya Y, Izawa H. Serial evaluation of human anterior cruciate ligament grafts by contrast-enhanced magnetic resonance imaging: comparison of allografts and autografts. Arthroscopy 2008;24(9):1038–44.
15. Harris NL, Indelicato PA, Bloomberg MS, et al. Radiographic and histologic analysis of the tibial tunnel after allograft anterior cruciate ligament reconstruction in goats. Am J Sports Med 2002;30(3):368–73.
16. Scheffler SU, Schmidt T, Gangey I, et al. Fresh-frozen free-tendon allografts versus autografts in anterior cruciate ligament reconstruction: delayed remodeling and inferior mechanical function during long-term healing in sheep. Arthroscopy 2008;24(4):448–58.
17. Edgar CM, Zimmer S, Kakar S, et al. Prospective comparison of auto and allograft hamstring tendon constructs for ACL reconstruction. Clin Orthop Relat Res 2008; 466(9):2238–46.
18. Harner CD, Olson E, Irrgang JJ, et al. Allograft versus autograft anterior cruciate ligament reconstruction: 3- to 5-year outcome. Clin Orthop Relat Res 1996;324: 134–44.
19. Indelicato PA, Bittar ES, Prevot TJ, et al. Clinical comparison of freeze-dried and fresh frozen patellar tendon allografts for anterior cruciate ligament reconstruction of the knee. Am J Sports Med 1990;18(4):335–42.
20. Poehling GG, Curl WW, Lee CA, et al. Analysis of outcomes of anterior cruciate ligament repair with 5-year follow-up: allograft versus autograft. Arthroscopy 2005;21(7):774–85.
21. Shelton WR, Treacy SH, Dukes AD, et al. Use of allografts in knee reconstruction: II. Surgical considerations. J Am Acad Orthop Surg 1998;6(3):169–75.
22. Shino K, Nakata K, Horibe S, et al. Quantitative evaluation after arthroscopic anterior cruciate ligament reconstruction. Allograft versus autograft. Am J Sports Med 1993;21(4):609–16.
23. Prodromos C, Joyce B, Shi K. A meta-analysis of stability of autografts compared to allografts after anterior cruciate ligament reconstruction. Knee Surg Sports Traumatol Arthrosc 2007;15(7):851–6.
24. Kaeding C, Pedroza A, Aros BC, et al. Independent predictors of ACL reconstruction failure from the MOON prospective longitudinal cohort. Presented at the AOSSM Annual Meeting; 2008.
25. Gross AE, McKee NH, Pritzker KP, et al. Reconstruction of skeletal deficits at the knee: a comprehensive osteochondral transplant program. Clin Orthop Relat Res 1983;174:96–106.
26. Gross AE, Silverstein EA, Falk J, et al. The allo-transplantation of partial joints in the treatment of osteoarthritis of the knee. Clin Orthop Relat Res 1975;108:7–14.
27. Langer F, Gross AE, West M, et al. The immunogenicity of allograft knee joint transplants. Clin Orthop Relat Res 1978;132:155–62.
28. McDermott AG, Langer F, Pritzker KP, et al. Fresh small-fragment osteochondral allografts. Long-term follow-up study on first 100 cases. Clin Orthop Relat Res 1985;(197):96–102.

29. Parrish FF. Allograft replacement of all or part of the end of a long bone following excision of a tumor. J Bone Joint Surg Am 1973;55:1–22.
30. Volkov M. Allotransplantation of joints. J Bone Joint Surg Am 1970;52:49–53.
31. Aubin PP, Cheah HK, Davis AM, et al. Long-term follow-up of fresh femoral osteochondral allografts for posttraumatic knee defects. Clin Orthop Relat Res 2001; 391(Suppl):S318–27.
32. Beaver RJ, Mahomed M, Backstein D, et al. Fresh osteochondral allografts for post-traumatic defects in the knee. A survivorship analysis 1992;74(1):105–10.
33. Buckwalter JA, Mankin HJ. Instructional course lectures, The American Academy of Orthopaedic Surgeons-articular cartilage. Part II: Degeneration and osteoarthritis, repair, regeneration, and transplantation. J Bone Joint Surg Am 1997;79: 612–32.
34. Lightfoot A, Martin J, Amendola A. Fluorescent viability stains overestimate chondrocyte viability in osteoarticular allografts. Am J Sports Med 2007;35(11): 1817–23.
35. Bugbee WD. Fresh osteochondral allografts. J Knee Surg 2002;15(3):191–5.
36. Gross AE, Kim W, Las Heras F, et al. Fresh osteochondral allografts for posttraumatic knee defects: long-term follow-up. Clin Orthop Relat Res 2008;466(8): 1863–70.
37. Williams RJ 3rd, Bugbee W, Convery F. Osteochondral allograft transplantation. Clin Sports Med 1999;18:67–75.
38. Allen RT, Robertson CM, Pennock AT, et al. Analysis of stored osteochondral allografts at the time of surgical implantation. Am J Sports Med 2005;33(10): 1479–84.
39. Ball ST, Amiel D, Williams SK, et al. The effects of storage on fresh human osteochondral allografts. Clin Orthop Relat Res 2004;418:246–52.
40. Rohde RS, Studer RK, Chu CR. Mini-pig fresh osteochondral allografts deteriorate after 1 week of cold storage. Clin Orthop Relat Res 2004;427:226–33.
41. Williams RJ 3rd, Dreese JC, Chen CT. Chondrocyte survival and material properties of hypothermically stored cartilage: an evaluation of tissue used for osteochondral allograft transplantation. Am J Sports Med 2004;32(1):132–9.
42. Marco F, Leon C, Lopez-Oliva F, et al. Intact articular cartilage cryopreservation. In vivo evaluation. Clin Orthop Relat Res 1992;283:11–20.
43. Ohlendorf C, Tomford WW, Mankin HJ. Chondrocyte survival in cryopreserved osteochondral articular cartilage. J Orthop Res 1996;14(3):413–6.
44. Pearsall AWIV, Tucker JA, Hester RB, et al. Chondrocyte viability in refrigerated osteochondral allografts used for transplantation within the knee. Am J Sports Med 2004;32(1):125–31.
45. Oates KM, Chen AC, Young EP, et al. Effect of tissue culture storage on the in vivo survival of canine osteochondral allografts. J Orthop Res 1995;13(4):562–9.
46. Malinin T, Temple HT, Buck BE. Transplantation of osteochondral allografts after cold storage. J Bone Joint Surg Am 2006;88(4):762–70.
47. Lubowitz JH, Verdonk PC, Reid JB 3rd, et al. Meniscus allograft transplantation: a current concepts review. Knee Surg Sports Traumatol Arthrosc 2007;15(5): 476–92.
48. Verdonk PC, Demurie A, Almqvist KF, et al. Transplantation of viable meniscal allograft. Survivorship analysis and clinical outcome of one hundred cases. J Bone Joint Surg Am 2005;87(4):715–24.
49. Alford W, Cole BJ. The indications and technique for meniscal transplant. Orthop Clin North Am 2005;36(4):469–84.

Primary ACL Reconstruction Using Allograft Tissue

J.C. Clark, MD[a],*, Daniel E. Rueff, MD[a],**, Peter A. Indelicato, MD[b],
Michael Moser, MD[c]

KEYWORDS

• Allograft processing • Allograft biology
• Achilles tendon allograft technique
• Tibialis anterior allograft technique
• Allograft clinical results

The use of allograft tissue in orthopedic surgery has increased substantially in the past several years. Take, for instance, the jump in the distribution of allografts from 350,000 in 1990 to 875,000 in 2001.[1] This number increased to more than 1 million in an estimate by the American Association of Tissue Banks (AATB) in 2004, and in 2006, approximately 1.5 million bone and tissue allografts were implanted throughout the United States.[2,3] About 10% of these were soft tissue allografts, which are commonly used in sports medicine procedures.[4] In fact, in a 2006 American Orthopaedic Society for Sports Medicine (AOSSM) survey of 365 respondents, 86% reported using allograft tissue in their practice.[5]

Consequently, the number of clinical and scientific reports that pepper the literature on the use of allografts has also exponentially increased. With such an influx of information, sorting it out can be time-consuming, intimidating, and downright confusing. This fact was exemplified by the same AOSSM survey mentioned earlier, in which 46% of the sample polled did not know whether the tissues they used were sterilized or the specific sterilization process used.[5] Moreover, 21% of the respondents did not know if their allografts came from AATB-accredited sources.[5]

This article focuses on the use of allograft for primary anterior cruciate ligament (ACL) reconstruction, including 2 techniques used by the senior authors at their institution. It is

Conflicts of Interest: Both Dr. Indelicato and Dr. Moser are consultants for Regeneration Technologies, Inc. (RTI).
[a] University of Florida Orthopaedic and Sports Medicine Institute, PO Box 112727, Gainesville, FL 32611, USA
[b] Sports Medicine, UF Athletic Association, University of Florida, Gainesville, FL, USA
[c] UF Athletic Association, University of Florida, Gainesville, FL, USA
* Corresponding author.
** Corresponding author.
E-mail addresses: clarkjc@ufl.edu (J. Clark); deruef01@ufl.edu (D.E. Rueff).

Clin Sports Med 28 (2009) 223–244
doi:10.1016/j.csm.2008.10.005
0278-5919/08/$ – see front matter © 2009 Elsevier Inc. All rights reserved.
sportsmed.theclinics.com

hoped that the reader will be able to come away with a greater understanding of allograft processing and preparation, risk of disease transmission, maturation after implantation, handling, and the clinical studies that support allograft use in ACL reconstruction.

ASPECTS OF ALLOGRAFT USE

Allografts are just one of the many options available for use in ACL reconstruction. There are several different allografts used today, including patellar tendon, quadriceps tendon, Achilles tendon, tibialis anterior tendon, tibialis posterior tendon, hamstring tendon, and fascia lata.[2] Currently, at the authors' institution, both Achilles tendon and tibialis anterior tendon allografts are used.

Allograft Processing

When discussing the use of allografts with patients, most are appropriately concerned about the possibility of disease transmission. To adequately answer a patient's questions about disease transmission, it is important for the surgeons to be familiar with the processes that their particular choice of allograft goes through before it arrives in the operating room.

Disease transmission can occur by several means. One method is the allograft contaminated from an infectious agent present in the donor's blood or body cavities at the time of death. This can occur from an occult perimortem infection, a screening failure, or possible dissemination of bowel cavity flora to the donor tissue.[5] The other method of transmission is contamination during harvesting, processing, and packaging.[5] Steps are taken during the various preparation techniques to avoid each of these modes of transmission.

Typically, before even harvesting or procurement can occur, the donor undergoes a rigorous screening, which includes a chart review, personal history from family members, and a rigorous physical examination to rule out high-risk behavior and potential communicable diseases. Blood and tissue tests are also performed to rule out infectious diseases like hepatitis and human immunodeficiency virus (HIV). Then, using aseptic procurement techniques and standard operating room protocol, the tissue is harvested, cultured, and often rinsed with an antimicrobial disinfectant before being wrapped, labeled, sealed, and sent to be formally sterilized. Although the tissues have been aseptically processed up to this point, they should not be considered sterile.

The goal of formal sterilization is to remove or inactivate microorganisms. Currently, primary sterilization is usually done by gamma irradiation (GI) and/or proprietary chemical processing.[2] The U.S. Food and Drug Administration (FDA) considers a sterility assurance level (SAL) of 10^{-3} as adequate (1 in 1000 chance that a living microbe exists) for implantation of biological medical devices.[5] Although beneficial with regard to removing and inactivating microorganisms, most current sterilization procedures carry the disadvantage of altering the biological properties and mechanical function of the allograft.[6-13] For example, it has been suggested by several studies that GI decreases allograft strength in a dose-dependent-manner.[11,14-18]

GI is a very effective sterilant, killing bacteria at doses of 1.5 to 2.5 Mrad, viruses and spores at >3.5 Mrad, and reaching an SAL of 10^{-6} at 8.9 mrad.[4] However, GI produces enough free radicals to substantially weaken collagen chains in allograft tissue around 3.0 Mrad.[4] To avoid this collagen destruction by GI, tissue banks favor a combined approach with chemical processing and lower levels of irradiation at around 1.0 to 3.5 Mrad, with the potential drawback of less inactivation of microorganisms. In the authors' own practice, irradiated grafts were abandoned after publication of the results for irradiated versus nonirradiated Achilles tendon allografts for primary ACL reconstruction by Rappe and colleagues[7] in 2007. In this series, there was a 33% versus 2.4% failure rate for irradiated versus nonirradiated allografts, respectively, using 2.0 to 2.5 Mrad of GI.

Currently, the allografts are formally sterilized by another type of primary sterilization technique, a proprietary low-temperature chemical processing procedure called BioCleanse (RTI Biologics, Alachua, FL). This system uses pressure variations to drive sterilants such as hydrogen peroxide and isopropyl alcohol into the tissue, achieving an SAL of 10^{-6}.[5] Other processes such as this are present throughout the United States. Each uses a different combination or series of cleansing, disinfection, and rinsing, with the ultimate goal of removing donor cells, microorganisms, and lipids. However, whether or not these chemical processing protocols can penetrate deep into the graft is a concern, which is why they are often followed by a terminal sterilization step. Ethylene oxide was once used for this step, but reports of synovitis, immune reactions, and graft dissolution led to its decline.[2] Most allografts, other than those processed via the BioCleanse technique, are now terminally sterilized with low-dose irradiation and then deep-frozen for storage until the time of surgery.

Chemical processing followed by irradiation is not the only sterilization method employed by tissue banks. Another process of sterilization is called *freeze-drying* or *lyophilization* in the literature. This process involves freezing the tissue, then subjecting it to several drying steps, the first being sublimation and the second being desorption. The allograft can then be stored at room temperature for up to 3 to 5 years and is rehydrated for 30 minutes before implantation. These steps can alter the mechanical properties of soft tissue allografts, which is why it is not commonly used in the United States for sports medicine.[5]

Aseptic fresh-frozen or deep-frozen allografts are those that are taken from a donor, cleansed with antibiotic soaks, and then typically frozen to less than $-80°C$. Although microorganisms, spores, and viruses such as HIV and hepatitis C can survive this process, sterility is presumably assured by proper donor selection, negative cultures, and serologic testing.[2] Immune reactions are avoided because donor cells are destroyed by the freezing process, thus decreasing antigenicity.

Risk of Disease Transmission

Despite all of this preparation, there is always a potential risk in transmitting disease using allografts, albeit lower than the risk with the transplantation of organs.[19] The U.S. Centers for Disease Control and Prevention (CDC) define an allograft-associated infection as one that occurs within 12 months of implantation in an otherwise healthy patient with no known risk factors.[4] In June 2002, the CDC reported a case of hepatitis C transmission from a patellar tendon allograft that was harvested in the year 2000.[20] This particular donor did not have an antibody to the hepatitis C virus (HCV) on the original serologic screening but subsequent nucleic acid testing (NAT) for HCV ribonucleic acid was positive. To avoid this problem of harvesting from a donor in a "window period," the surgeon should insist that his/her allografts be NAT tested. This may not be a problem for some surgeons who get allografts from FDA-regulated tissue banks, because now guidelines from the FDA require tissues distributed after August 2007 to be NAT tested and found HIV and HCV negative.[5] Although no definite number can be given for the absolute risk of HIV or hepatitis from soft tissue allografts, the estimated number for HIV and hepatitis is somewhere between 1 in 1 million and 1 in 1.6 million.[21–24] With regard to HIV, there have been no documented cases of viral transmission since 1995, when standards were placed regarding more thorough testing of donor and allograft. Before 1995, there were 8 reported cases of musculoskeletal allograft-associated HIV infection.[1,25,26] To put this in perspective, the risk of someone aged 15 to 24 years dying from an unintentional injury such as a motor vehicle accident in 2005 was 37.4/100,000, the risk of suicide was 10/100,000, and the risk of homicide was 13/100,000.[27] Despite these numbers, the repercussions felt by both patient and physician if transmission occurs can be devastating.

The risk of bacterial infection from allograft tissue is unknown at this point. However, no difference in the rate of septic arthritis after autograft and allograft ACL reconstruction has been reported.[28] Nonetheless, bacterial transmission in allograft surgery was highlighted in 2000 when several patients receiving BPTB allografts developed septic arthritis.[4,29] Shortly thereafter, in 2001, concern with allograft-associated infections peaked with the death of a recipient of a femoral condyle allograft contaminated with *Clostridium sordellii*.[30] The subsequent CDC investigation in 2002 of 26 allograft-associated bacterial infections found a *Clostridium septicum and Clostridium sordellii* species to be the cause in half of the infections. Most importantly to sports medicine specialists, the majority of these allografts were hemipatellar tendons for ACL reconstructions.[31] Recommendations for more stringent sporicidal tissue processing as well as avoidance of a prolonged interval between death and harvesting were made, during which time bowel flora can hematogenously spread throughout the body.[32,33] Unfortunately, most of these cases were associated with a single tissue bank but had the effect of eroding the population's confidence about allografts. Despite the heightened awareness, bacterial infections have still been reported since then, including a 17-year-old patient who developed a *Streptococcus pyogenes* septic arthritis after allograft ACL reconstruction.[34]

These reports led to several articles being published about culturing allograft tissue at the time of implantation. Diaz-de-Rada and colleagues[35] cultured BPTB allografts in 181 patients and obtained 24 positive cultures (13.26%). Patients with positive allograft cultures were treated with 2 weeks of oral antibiotics after surgery. Clinical signs of infection did not develop in these patients acutely, but final long-term follow-up was not reported. Guelich and colleagues[1] found that 24 of 247 (9.7%) Achilles tendon or tibialis anterior tendon allografts had positive cultures after implantation. None of these patients received anything more than the standard preoperative and postoperative prophylactic antibiotics. At an average of 7.5 months after surgery, none of the patients with a positive allograft culture had evidence of infection.[1] Publications such as this prompted a workshop in June 2005 titled "Preventing Organ and Tissue Allograft-Transmitted Infection: Priorities for Public Health Intervention" (Blood, Organ, and Other Tissues Safety [BOOTS] Workshop) to suggest that culturing of allografts was not appropriate before implantation in the operating room if they were sterilized or aseptically processed with negative final cultures from the tissue bank.[5] At the authors' institution, no routine cultures of allografts are performed before implantation.

Prion infections, such as Jakob-Cruetzfeldt disease, have raised concern as well, because there is a lack of validated screening tests for these types of infections. Thus, the risk of acquiring these infections from allografts is unknown but likely low because of their overall low prevalence. Unfortunately, prion infections may take more than 10 years to manifest, so future reports may surface.

Advantages/Disadvantages of Allograft

The proposed advantages of using allografts for primary ACL reconstruction include a lack of donor-site morbidity, unlimited available sizes, shorter operative times, availability of larger grafts, smaller incisions, improved cosmesis, lower incidence of postoperative arthrofibrosis, faster immediate postoperative recovery, and less postoperative pain.[1,36–38]

Classically, the disadvantages of allograft are mainly concerned with potential disease transmission, as mentioned earlier, and prolonged graft healing necessitating a delay in return to competition. However, newer concerns have risen such as a lower normal stability rate and higher failure rate based on meta-analytic data pooling of KT-1000 measurements by Prodromos and colleagues[39] at a minimum 2-year follow-up. Whether these stability rates change to those at which autografts and allografts approach one another is not understood, but several reports concerning further increases in allograft failure rates have been published.[40–42]

The use of allograft tissue has also been thought to result in a financial loss for hospitals and surgery centers. However, Cole and colleagues[43] showed allograft use to be less costly when comparing freeze-dried Achilles tendon to BPTB autograft. One of the main reasons for the autograft being more expensive was the increased operating room time and high hospitalization rates after autograft.

In general, the issue of cost will primarily depend on the institution and surgery center. For patient counseling, surgeons should be familiar with the relative cost of allograft versus autograft in their own practice, because this may ultimately make the decision for the patient.

Biologic Incorporation of Allograft

Autografts and allografts undergo a similar sequence of biologic events for both incorporation into host bone tunnels and ligamentization of the intra-articular portion.[44–47] Within the graft substance itself, this involves graft necrosis with degeneration, an inflammatory response, cellular repopulation of the graft scaffold, revascularization, and finally graft healing and remodeling as the collagen becomes more organized. Tunnel healing involves either bone-to-bone healing, bone-to-tendon healing, or a combination of the 2 depending on the type of graft used. Typically, for autografts, tendon-to-bone healing is considered to occur slower (8–12 weeks) than bone-to-bone healing (6 weeks).[48] The same can be said for allograft bone tunnel healing. In a study by one of the authors (PAI), BPTB allograft incorporation into tibial tunnels was shown to be complete at 18 weeks, with formation of fibrous tissue between the graft and tunnel wall.[49]

The publications on allograft ligamentization that most timelines of allograft maturation are derived from warrant mention. Arnoczky showed that deep-frozen patellar tendon allografts in dogs were well perfused at 6 to 8 weeks with an area of central hypovascularity that persisted until 3 to 4 months.[50] Revascularization was complete by 6 months and the gross and histologic appearance similar to that of a normal ACL by 1 year.

In a goat model, Jackson compared similar-sized patellar tendon autografts and fresh-frozen allografts.[46] Although at time zero the mechanical and structural properties were equivalent, the 6-month mark revealed a statistically significant difference in favor of autografts with regard to anterior-posterior displacement and maximal load to failure. Histologically, allografts had a prolonged inflammatory response and diminished cross-sectional area growth between the 6-week and 6-month interval compared with autografts. Autografts had an increased and more robust density of small-diameter collagen fibrils and increased cross-sectional area at 6 months. In the bone tunnels, both grafts showed similar histology of bone plug incorporation and tendon-bone healing.

Shino and colleagues[51] examined biopsy specimens of deep-frozen allografts in humans taken during arthroscopy at 3 to 55 months after transplantation. They concluded that full graft maturity was not reached until 18 months, although by 12 months they looked like normal ACLs macroscopically. In a previous study by Shino using the canine, he compared deep-frozen patellar tendon allograft with autograft.[52] In this study, allograft had the same mechanical properties as autograft after 30 weeks. After 52 weeks, the allograft had a histologic appearance similar to that of a normal ACL.

Also using the canine model, Nikolaou and colleagues compared autograft versus cryopreserved allograft at 8, 16, 24, 36, and 78 weeks.[53] Macroscopically, the allograft was indistinguishable from the normal control ACL at 36 weeks. The histologic and microangiographic appearance of autografts at 16 weeks was almost normal, whereas it was almost normal for allografts at 24 weeks. At 18 months, allograft specimens had both a completely normal collagen and vascular framework with complete replacement of the graft by host cells. Biomechanical evaluation showed that the allograft was similar to autograft at the 36-week mark but lagged behind autograft strength up to that point.

In a unique study and one of the first of its kind, Malinin and coworkers described the histology of retrieved frozen or freeze-dried allografts from 20 days to 10 years after transplantation.[54] Their findings suggest an even slower maturation process than that postulated by Shino and point out that maturation of the allograft within the joint appears to be faster than maturation within the bone tunnels. Although the entire allograft becomes revascularized and replaced with host cells, it is not uniform according to this study and may not be complete until 3 years or longer. Particularly within the tunnel, thin rims of newly formed cortical bone were found in the 3.5-year specimens but not in the 2-year specimens. Interestingly, the one autograft that was retrieved and compared with an allograft of the same age (2 years) had a similar appearance both within the joint and within the tunnels. In a similar, but separate, case report study by Lee and coworkers, a freeze-dried Achilles tendon allograft was retrieved at the time of knee replacement 2.5 years after ACL reconstruction.[55] The authors described full cellularity of the graft and normal crimp pattern. In the tibial tunnel, the allograft showed Sharpey's fibers where the graft inserted into the tibial bone.

More recently, in a sheep model study, autograft and allograft flexor digitorum superficialis tendons were used for ACL reconstruction.[56] The animals were studied at 6, 12, and 52 weeks. At the 6-week mark, the allografts showed lower overall cellularity and vascularity than autografts. This situation reversed at 12 weeks, with allograft showing more cellularity, albeit less homogenous and with more hypocellular areas, especially at the center of the allograft. Vascular density was still less in allografts at this stage. Essentially, the histologic appearance of allografts at 12 weeks was similar to the histologic appearance of autografts at 6 weeks. By 52 weeks, both the allograft's and autograft's cellular and vascular patterns closely resembled the normal control ACL's patterns. Interestingly, despite the histologic differences, biomechanical testing showed no significant difference between allograft and autograft tendon at 6 and 12 weeks. However, at 52 weeks, AP laxity was larger and the stress, stiffness, and failure loads were lower for the allograft group.

One of the most important points that can be gleaned from the above-mentioned studies is that allografts undergo a maturation process similar to that of autografts, although in a delayed fashion. The time to full maturation and complete remodeling of the allograft without any further change in histology is unknown at this time although it is possibly longer than a year. Despite the delayed maturation shown in these laboratory models, the clinical outcomes of allograft ACL reconstruction appear similar to those of autograft.

ACHILLES TENDON ALLOGRAFT TECHNIQUE (P.A.I.)
Patient Selection

Allograft ACL reconstruction is offered to all patients with acute, chronic, or failed ACL tears regardless of age. The trend is to perform hamstring autograft ACL reconstruction on patients younger than 14 years and use allograft on everyone else. Before deciding which graft to use, the patient goes through the standard informed consent process and financial counseling on autograft versus allograft. If allograft is chosen, a specific separate consent is signed regarding the risk of infection from allograft, including hepatitis and HIV transmission. For this technique, the senior author uses nonirradiated BioCleanse Achilles tendon allograft (RTI Biologics, Alachua, FL) with a bone plug (**Fig. 1**).

Patient Preparation

At the preoperative visit, the patient is given instructions on how to perform an antimicrobial soap scrub of the operative site the night before surgery and then the morning of the surgery before coming to the ambulatory surgery suite. When the patient arrives to the preoperative area, the operative site is identified by the nurse, shaven with electric clippers, and then marked by the orthopaedic service. As the patient gets into the operating room, a time-out is done with the attending anesthesiologist and then a second time-out is done with the attending surgeon before prepping and draping begin. Once the patient is properly anesthetized, Lachman and pivot shift tests are performed, along with testing of the medial collateral ligament (MCL), lateral collateral ligament (LCL), posterior cruciate ligament (PCL), and posterolateral corner to rule out any associated injuries. A nonsterile tourniquet is placed high on the thigh with cast padding underneath. A thigh post is then placed one hand-breadth proximal to the superior pole of the patella to aid in the diagnostic arthroscopy portion of the procedure. All the patients are then prepped with chlorhexidine scrub and draped with a combination of stockinet, down drapes, plastic U-drapes, an extremity drape, and elastic bandage wrapped around the lower leg. Finally, a hole is cut in the stockinet to expose the knee. While the scrub technician is setting up the arthroscopy equipment, the orthopedic team prepares the graft on the back table.

Graft Preparation

Before arthroscopy is performed, the graft is made ready on a sterile back table. The graft has already been thawed in a saline, bacitracin, and polymyxin B solution by the scrub technician. Typically, this takes about 20 minutes. Once thawed, the graft is inspected for defects and quality of tissue (**Fig. 2**). The bone plug is rongeured to around 20 mm long and the tip is shaped like a bullet to allow easier entry into the femoral canal. A 2-mm drill hole is then made in the bone plug to accommodate the passage of 2 No. 5 Ticron sutures (Sherwood, Davis & Geck, St. Louis, MO). Sizing of the bone plug is then done, with measurements typically falling in the 10-mm diameter range. This allows one to get the drills ready for the tibial and femoral tunnels,

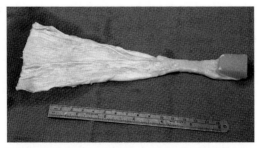

Fig. 1. Nonirradiated BioCleanse Achilles tendon allograft. The bone plug is fashioned from this block shape into a bullet shape for easier passage through the tunnels.

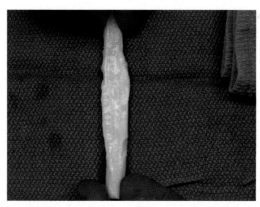

Fig. 2. Example of an allograft with poor tissue quality and poor preparation. Note the yellow areas within the graft consisting of fatty tissue.

which are drilled 1 mm wider than the bone plug diameter. While an assistant holds the sutures passing through the bone plug, a Krackow-type stitch is done through the tendinous portion of the graft with a No. 5 Ticron suture. A marking pen is used to draw a line circumferentially at the bone plug–tendon junction for later identification when placing the graft in the femoral tunnel. The graft is then placed on a tensioning board at 20 lb tension with a wet lap wrapped around it to prevent desiccation (**Fig. 3**).

Arthroscopy

A standard diagnostic arthroscopy is performed first by examining the patellofemoral joint and then the medial and lateral compartments. The intercondylar notch is inspected, and the ACL tear is confirmed with visualization and probing. Any repairable meniscal tears or other intra-articular abnormalities are addressed at this time.

The native ACL is taken down with an arthroscopic oscillating shaver, and the insertion on the tibial plateau is defined with an arthroscopic wand. Then the wand is used to expose the notch by subperiosteally elevating all synovium and ACL remnants from anterior to posterior off the medial side of the lateral femoral condyle. The notchplasty is done with an arthroscopic aggressive shaver, taking around 5 to 10 mm of bone from the lateral femoral condyle's medial side. However, varying amounts of bone are taken depending on the patient's particular notch anatomy. The goal is to adequately visualize the posterior notch for placement of the femoral tunnel and provide enough room for the allograft.

Graft Placement

Once the notch has been prepared, a curved curette is used to mark the over-the-top position. This allows one to better visualize the entrance of the femoral tunnel, which is

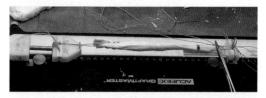

Fig. 3. Prepared allograft on the tensioning board. A Krackow-type stitch has been placed through the tendinous portion and several nonabsorbable sutures placed through the bone plug.

then marked with the curette and deepened with the arthroscopic shaver. The entrance is preferred to be about 6 mm anterior to the posterior cortex and at the 10 o'clock position for a right knee (**Fig. 4**).

Attention is then directed to the tibial tunnel. With the scope in the lateral parapatellar portal, the ACL footprint is visualized as the ACL guide is brought through the medial portal and placed in the appropriate position in the ACL footprint. Once it is in position, the skin is marked with the guide and a 2-cm incision is made over the mark hard to bone and perpendicular to the anteromedial face of the tibia. Care is taken to make the majority of the incision superior to the skin mark to prevent stretching of the skin while drilling. A guide pin is then drilled through the ACL guide and into the joint, watching with the scope for penetration through the plateau. The position of the guide wire is checked and then a cannulated straight reamer is used to make the tibial tunnel. The reamer and tibial guide pin are then withdrawn, and a cannulated bone tunnel plug is inserted into the hole in the tibia. An arthroscopic shaver is inserted through the plug and used to clear any bony debris and smooth the tibial tunnel edges. A 2.4-mm diameter trocar-tipped passing pin (Beath pin) is inserted through the tibial tunnel and into the previously identified femoral starting point on the posterolateral notch. This passing pin is drilled through the femur and out the skin of the lateral thigh. Since an EndoButton (Smith & Nephew, Memphis, TN) is used for femoral fixation, the femoral tunnel is then drilled with the 4.5-mm EndoButton reamer over the passing pin and through the lateral femoral cortex. While reaming, attention is paid to the depth on the reamer before plunging through the cortex to get an estimate of femoral tunnel length. This is typically around 40 mm (**Fig. 5**). An acorn reamer is then inserted and the femoral tunnel is drilled, avoiding penetration of the lateral femoral cortex. If the lateral femoral cortex is breached, an Extendobutton (Smith & Nephew, Memphis, TN) is used to increase the diameter of the button.

Once the femoral tunnel is drilled, the knee is irrigated to remove any debris from the drilling. A No. 5 Ethibond (Ethicon, Somerville, NJ) passing suture is pulled through the knee and out the skin of the lateral thigh with the passing pin. The edges of the femoral tunnel are chamfered, especially anteriorly, with an arthroscopic shaver. A depth

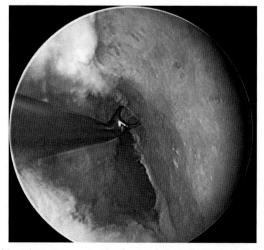

Fig. 4. Curette marking the entrance to the femoral tunnel. For the left knee, this is typically at the 2 o'clock position and 6 to 7 mm anterior to the posterior cortex.

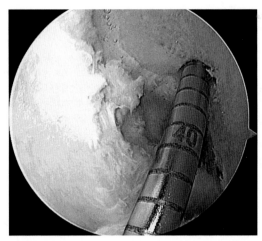

Fig. 5. The reamer for the EndoButton (Smith & Nephew, Memphis, TN) is passed over the passing pin and drilled through the lateral cortex of the femur. The reamer is about to go through the cortex in this picture, so an estimated femoral tunnel length can be obtained.

gauge is then inserted up through the tibial tunnel to measure the length of the femoral tunnel more precisely.

Graft Fixation

Using an EndoButton for femoral fixation and a fully threaded bioabsorbable interference screw (Bio-Interference, Arthrex, Naples, FL) for tibial fixation in the tibial tunnel is preferred. Additional fixation is achieved with a 5.5 mm × 18.3 mm PEEK-OPTIMA SwiveLock Screw (Arthrex, Naples, FL). Based on the measurement of the femoral tunnel length, an appropriate EndoButton is chosen. The long loop of the EndoButton is passed through the previously drilled hole in the bone plug. Next, 2 different colored No. 5 Ethibond sutures are passed through the metal holes in the EndoButton. With an assistant, the graft and EndoButton system are tensioned. Once the graft is prepared, the 2 different colored sutures are passed through the tibia, joint, and femoral tunnel using the passing suture already in place. The different colored sutures allow one to be sure that the EndoButton is pulled up through the femoral tunnel in a lengthwise position with a leading suture. It is then deployed with the lagging suture, and the button is toggled on the lateral femoral cortex several times to seat it on the lateral femoral cortex. Pulling the EndoButton up with both sutures simultaneously may result in it becoming incarcerated in the femoral tunnel. With femoral fixation in place, the leg is then placed into extension on top of the table for tensioning of the graft and insertion of the tibial interference screw using a guide wire. After tibial fixation is complete, a PEEK-OPTIMA SwiveLock Screw is used for additional fixation of the free suture ends from the graft. Any redundant allograft tissue and suture are cut with a knife. A Lachman's test is then performed to assure a well-functioning graft. A drain is placed into the joint through one of the portals, and a subcutaneous drain is placed in the medial tibial wound exiting superiorly. Bupivacaine 0.25% with epinephrine is injected into the joint and into the tissue surrounding the medial tibial incision and the portal sites. Portal sites are closed with simple sutures, and the medial tibial wound is closed in typical layered fashion (**Fig. 6**). Sterile dressings are applied and wrapped with soft cast padding, a Cryocuff, elastic bandage wraps, and a knee immobilizer.

Immediate Postoperative Care and Rehabilitation

Patients are seen on the first postoperative day. During this visit, drains are removed, the knee is passively ranged, and dressing changes are taught to the patient and family. Then, the patient goes immediately to physical therapy where the ACL rehabilitation protocol is thoroughly discussed and initiated. The entire protocol is divided into 6 phases with criteria-based progression through the protocol. Generally, independent straight running does not begin until week 12 as long as criteria have been met, particularly strength and range of motion. Patients are not allowed to return to sport until achieving full range of motion, completion of an agility and sport-specific program, strength approaches >85% of the opposite leg based on Biodex testing (Biodex Medical Systems, Inc., New York, NY), KT-2000 testing shows <3 mm side-to-side difference, and no effusion is present. It has been found that this occurs around 6 months postoperatively.

TIBIALIS ANTERIOR TENDON ALLOGRAFT TECHNIQUE (M.M.)
Graft Selection

A non-irradiated BioCleanse tibialis anterior tendon (RTI Biologics, Alachua, FL) is the preferred allograft of the senior author for this technique. There are several reasons why this graft is chosen. Doubled tibialis anterior grafts have been found to have the highest tensile strength and stiffness of all commonly used grafts for ACL reconstruction.[57] Unlike an Achilles tendon or BPTB allograft, a tibialis anterior allograft is entirely soft tissue, allowing easier graft passage and eliminating the requirement to fashion a bone plug. Additionally, there is no need to rely on the frequently soft

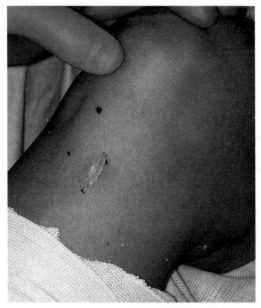

Fig. 6. Two centimeter incision before closure. This tibial incision and 3 portal sites are the only incisions used during allograft ACL reconstruction for this (senior author's) technique.

bone comprising the bone plug for graft fixation, and the thin bone plug–soft tissue junction is avoided. Finally, soft tissue grafts allow for a larger diameter graft with more complete fill of the bone tunnel compared with BPTB or Achilles tendon allografts.

Patient Selection

For primary ACL reconstruction, the senior surgeon (M.M.) uses both autograft hamstring and allograft tibialis anterior tendon grafts. Tibialis anterior tendon allografts are preferred in the majority of patients due to the decreased postoperative pain and morbidity, quicker surgical time, and better cosmesis. Exceptions would include younger patients (<25 years old) or high-level athletes due to the slower graft incorporation and bone-tendon healing compared with autograft tissues, which could delay return to sport.[45,58,59] However, at the authors' institution, tibialis anterior allografts have been used with good outcomes in all patient demographics in both primary and revision ACL reconstructions as well as multi-ligamentous knee injuries.

Patient Positioning

The patient undergoes the same preoperative assessment and preparation before coming back to the operating room as the previous senior author's patients. They are offered a regional block preoperatively and then placed on the operating table in the supine position. General anesthesia via a laryngeal mask airway is administered, and the injured and contralateral knees are examined. Range of motion as well as examination for ligamentous instability is performed including Lachman's test, anterior and posterior drawer, pivot shift, varus/valgus laxity, and posterolateral instability. Once the diagnosis of ACL insufficiency is confirmed, the allograft is opened and thawed on the back table by placing it into a solution of normal saline, bacitracin, and polymyxin B at room temperature. A nonsterile tourniquet is applied to the upper thigh and a small bump placed under the midthigh to allow increased knee flexion during the procedure. The knee is then prepped and draped in routine fashion. Antibiotics are administered, the leg is elevated and exsanguinated, and the tourniquet is insufflated.

Graft Preparation

While the diagnostic knee arthroscopy is being performed, the graft is prepared on the back table. The allograft is completely thawed before manipulating the graft to prevent damaging the tissue. The graft is then examined to evaluate its quality and survey for any structural defects, which would weaken its strength. Rarely, the graft will not meet the surgeon's standards and will need to be substituted with a new graft. A No. 2 Ticron suture (Sherwood, Davis & Geck, St. Louis, MO) is whip-stitched into the thinner proximal musculotendinous end of the graft for approximately 20 mm. A No. 5 Ticron suture is weaved through the thicker tendinous distal end of the graft. The edges of each end of the graft are then tapered with a knife to allow easier passage through the tunnels, the graft is folded upon itself, and the diameter is measured. The grafts can range from 8 to 10 mm, although they usually measure 9 mm. Measuring graft diameter at this point allows the scrub technician to prepare the proper drills for creating the tunnels. The drill diameter usually corresponds to the size of the graft or is 1 mm larger, ensuring easy passage of the graft. The doubled graft is placed on a tensioning board at 20 lbs and covered with a moist lap sponge (**Fig. 7**).

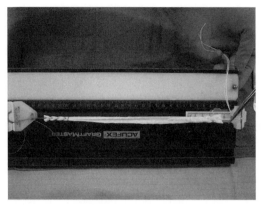

Fig. 7. Tibialis anterior tendon allograft on a tensioning board after Ticron sutures are whip-stitched at each end.

Arthroscopy

While the graft is being prepared, a diagnostic arthroscopy to evaluate for any articular or meniscal pathology is performed. The ACL tear is confirmed, the remnants are debrided, and meniscal injuries are addressed.

Next, the lateral post is removed, the knee is flexed to 90°, and a notchplasty is performed. The resection is performed with an arthroscopic shaver, starting anteriorly and proceeding back to the posterior cortex. The roof and lateral wall are resected just enough to prevent impingement of the graft through a full range of motion and to provide exposure of the lateral wall and over-the-top position (**Fig. 8**). A curette is used to mark the starting point for the femoral tunnel. Ideally, this allows for 1 to 2 mm of posterior tunnel wall at the 10 o'clock position for the right knees and the 2 o'clock position for the left knees.

Tunnel Creation

The arthroscopic tibial guide is set to 50° and inserted through the medial portal. The tip is placed at the posterior aspect of the ACL tibial footprint in line with the posterior

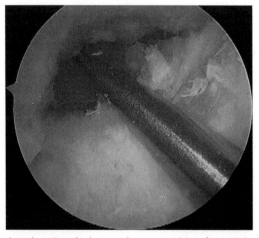

Fig. 8. Probe evaluating the 10 o'clock over-the-top position for a right knee.

border of the anterior horn of the lateral meniscus. It should be positioned as medial as possible while ensuring not to ream the medial tibial plateau. A 2-cm longitudinal incision is made in the middle of the anteromedial face of the tibia, 2 to 3 cm medial to the tibial tubercle. The periosteum is incised, and the tibial guide is positioned on the anterior cortex. The guide pin is advanced into the tibia and visualized arthroscopically as it enters the joint, confirming accurate positioning. The guide is removed, and the tibial reamer is drilled over the pin and visualized as it enters the joint. The guide pin is then removed, and the femoral reamer is pushed by hand into the previously marked starting location for the femoral tunnel on the lateral wall of the notch.

Femoral fixation is provided by an EndoButton CL Ultra (Smith & Nephew, Memphis, TN). The femoral reamer is advanced but stopped before penetrating the lateral cortex, usually correlating to a tunnel length of 35 to 45 mm. To provide at least 20 mm of graft-to-bone tunnel contact, the femoral socket must measure a minimum of 30 mm in length to allow for the EndoButton device to be deployed. If the cortex is encountered before 30 mm, it is breeched with the tunnel reamer and fixation is provided by an Extendobutton (Smith & Nephew, Memphis, TN). When drilling of the femoral tunnel is finished, the drill is removed, and the 4.5 mm EndoButton reamer is placed into the femoral tunnel and drilled out the lateral cortex. The depth gauge is inserted and the tunnel measured. The openings of the tibial and femoral tunnels are chamfered to prevent graft impingement.

Graft Passage and Fixation

A passing pin (Beath pin) is inserted through the tibial and femoral tunnels and pushed out through the skin. A looped No. 2 Ticron suture is attached to the distal end of the passing pin and pulled through the tunnels to later act as a passing suture. At the back table, the continuous loop of the EndoButton is affixed to the closed end of the doubled graft, and a white No. 5 Ticron suture and blue No. 2 Ticron suture are attached to holes in the EndoButton (**Fig. 9**). A reference line is placed on the graft at the location it will exit the femoral tunnel when seated and 10 mm distal to this mark corresponding to the extra length needed to flip the EndoButton. The passing suture is then used to pass the EndoButton sutures through the tunnels. Under arthroscopic visualization, tension is applied to the sutures (white first, then blue to pull up slack), and the graft is advanced to the pre-marked line. The EndoButton is deployed

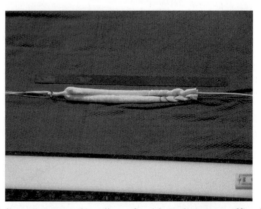

Fig. 9. Doubled tibialis anterior tendon allograft with EndoButton affixed and prepared for tunnel passage.

by pulling on the lagging suture and then firmly seated by applying tension to the sutures in a back and forth motion.

The distal graft sutures are pulled firmly to ensure that the EndoButton has been fully seated (**Fig. 10**). The knee is brought into full extension while visualizing arthroscopically for any notch impingement on the graft (**Fig. 11**). A BioRCI bioabsorbable interference screw (Smith & Nephew, Memphis, TN) equal to or 1 mm larger than the size of the tibial tunnel and 25 mm in length is selected, based on the quality of the bone. With the leg placed in 20° of flexion, the interference screw guide wire is placed anterior to the graft. The interference screw is advanced slowly through the tibial tunnel while pulling tension on the graft sutures and applying a posterior force to the tibia. The screw tip is advanced to the proximal end of the tibial tunnel, stopping just before entering the joint. No backup fixation is routinely used. A Lachman's test is performed to confirm the stability of the construct.

A drain is placed in the knee through a portal and the tibial wound closed in layered fashion with a running subcuticular closure for the skin. Simple sutures are used for the portal incisions and 0.25% bupivacaine is injected into the portal sites and intra-articularly. A sterile dressing, elastic bandages, Cryocuff, and knee immobilizer are placed in routine fashion.

Immediate Postoperative Care and Rehabilitation

Weight bearing is allowed in patients as tolerated on crutches. They are seen the first day postoperatively in the clinic, where their dressing is changed, the drain is removed, and physical therapy is initiated. The rehabilitation program is as described in the section on Achilles allograft reconstructions.

CLINICAL RESULTS FOR ALLOGRAFT ACL RECONSTRUCTION

There have been numerous studies evaluating the outcomes of allograft ACL reconstructions and their comparisons to autograft reconstructions. The literature has demonstrated successful outcomes with allograft use and most studies have shown little difference when comparing allograft and autograft reconstructions.[39,40,48,60–66] However, difficulty is encountered when comparing the various reconstruction

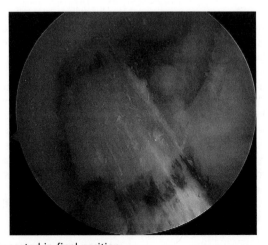

Fig. 10. Graft firmly seated in final position.

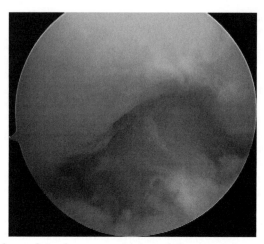

Fig. 11. Evaluating for graft impingement with knee fully extended.

methods due to the variety of graft tissues, surgical techniques, clinical outcome measures, and rehabilitation protocols used in the studies.

Several authors have reported their clinical outcomes with allograft ACL reconstructions. Noyes reported on 68 patients at mean follow-up of 7 years who had undergone acute ACL reconstruction with either a fascia lata (59%) or BPTB (41%) allograft.[60] KT-1000 examination demonstrated that 79% of the knees had less than a 3 mm side-to-side difference compared with the contralateral limb. The overall results were found to be excellent or good in 66% of the patients, and the graft failure rate was 14%. Noyes recommended reconstruction with a BPTB autogenous graft as the first choice for an acute ACL rupture but demonstrated that successful outcomes can be obtained with allograft tissue.

Nyland and coworkers retrospectively reviewed the results of 18 patients at 2 years after ACL reconstruction with cryopreserved tibialis anterior allografts.[61] Manual knee ligament tests demonstrated that 94% of knees were found to have normal or near-normal examinations, and KT-1000 measurements revealed an average 2 mm increase during maximum force testing of the involved side. All subjects continued to participate at their pre-injury perceived activity level. Nyland found ACL reconstruction with tibialis anterior allografts an effective alternative for older individuals and a promising surgical option for younger athletic patients who place higher loads across the knee joint.

In 2008, Nakata and colleagues[62] reported on the long-term outcomes (mean, 11.5 years) of 61 young active patients (mean, 20.9 years) who underwent ACL reconstruction using fresh-frozen tendon allograft with Achilles, tibialis anterior, or posterior tibialis tendons. Subjectively, 99% of patients graded their knees as normal or nearly normal. KT-2000 showed that 92% of patients had less than 3 mm side-to-side difference. The authors concluded that ACL reconstruction with soft tissue allografts can result in long-term knee stabilization among young active individuals while avoiding graft-harvest-site morbidity.

Other studies have demonstrated less successful outcomes with allograft reconstruction, with poor results due to factors such as graft sources, sterilization techniques, or rehabilitation protocols. Sterling reviewed the results of 18 patients who underwent ACL reconstruction with freeze-dried, ethylene oxide–sterilized BPTB allografts.[63] There were 6 graft failures (33%) noted at final follow-up. The authors recommended against ethylene oxide sterilization of grafts and concluded that a long shelf life negatively affects graft integrity.

Singhal and coworkers[58] retrospectively reviewed 125 patients who underwent ACL reconstruction with a tibialis anterior tendon allograft and an accelerated rehabilitation protocol. At mean follow-up of 55 months, 16 patients (23%) required revision for graft failure.

The mean age at which failure occurred was 22.8 years compared with 34 years in those in whom failure did not occur. The authors did not recommend using tibialis anterior allografts and an accelerated rehabilitation protocol in young or older active patients.

When directly comparing allograft with autograft ACL reconstructions, most studies have shown comparable outcomes. Harner[64] and associates reported on a retrospective study comparing 64 patients who underwent ACL reconstruction with nonirradiated allograft tissue with 26 patients who underwent reconstruction using autograft tissue at 3- to 5-year follow-up. Overall outcome based on International Knee Documentation Committee (IKDC) evaluation was normal or nearly normal in 48% of the allograft patients and 38% of the autograft group. No significant differences were found except a greater loss of terminal extension in the autograft patients (3°) than in the allograft patients (1.2°). The authors concluded that allograft tissue for ACL reconstruction is an acceptable alternative to autograft sources.

Peterson and colleagues[65] performed a prospective nonrandomized study comparing allograft versus autograft BPTB ACL reconstructions (30 patients in each group) at an average of 63 months. There was 1 graft failure in each group, and there were no differences in pain, giving way, effusion, Lachman's test, pivot shift test results, or KT-1000 measurements. The autograft group was found to have a significantly higher terminal extension loss (2.47°) than that of the allograft group (1.07°). The authors concluded that ACL reconstruction with BPTB autografts or allografts produced similar results and that allograft is an acceptable choice for ACL reconstruction.

In contrast, Chang[40] and associates reported on less successful outcomes with allograft ACL reconstruction. In a retrospective review, 46 allograft BPTB and 33 autograft BPTB ACL reconstructions were followed for a minimum of 2 years. All reconstructions were augmented with an iliotibial band tenodesis. There were no significant differences between groups in KT-1000 side-to-side differences, Lysholm II scores, or in any subjective category. More allograft patients complained of retropatellar pain (16% versus 9% for autograft patients), and 53% of allograft patients versus 23% of autograft patients had a flexion deficit of 5° or more. There were 3 traumatic ruptures in the allograft group (6.5%) and none in the autograft group. The authors concluded that allograft ACL reconstructions were comparable, but not equal, to autograft BPTB ACL reconstructions. Though allografts are a reasonable alternative, autograft BPTB reconstructions should remain the gold standard.

A retrospective study by Stringham and colleagues evaluated the outcomes of 47 BPTB autografts versus 31 BPTB allograft ACL reconstructions at 34 months' follow-up.[66] No significant differences were found between the groups when evaluating Lysholm scores, Tegner activity scores, patellofemoral symptoms, KT-1000 data, or isokinetic results. Traumatic graft failures occurred in 4 allograft patients compared with no traumatic ruptures in the autograft group. The authors concluded that autografts were their first choice for ACL reconstructions due to the higher traumatic failure in allograft patients.

In 2007, Prodromos and coworkers[39] reported the results of the first meta-analysis comparing the stability rates of autografts and allografts in ACL reconstruction. Using strict inclusion criteria (arthrometric follow-up data using at least 30 lb or maximum manual force, stratified presentation of stability data, and minimum 2-year follow-up), 20 allograft series were selected and compared with a previously published data set of all BPTB and hamstring autograft series. Allografts had significantly lower normal stability rates (59%) than autografts (72%). The allograft abnormal stability rate, usually representing graft failure, was significantly higher (14%) than that of autografts (5%). The authors concluded that the literature shows allograft ACL reconstruction to have substantially lower stability rates than those with autografts. The exact reasons for this lower performance are unclear but probably involved factors such as immunologic response, freezing, lack of cryopreservation, increased donor age, increased graft shelf time, subclinical infection, and radiation sterilization.

SUMMARY

ACL reconstruction has become one of the most common procedures performed by orthopedic surgeons with nearly 300,000 carried out in the United States each year.[2] While BPTB autograft continues to be the "gold standard" and most popular graft choice, the use of allograft tissues in ACL reconstruction has steadily increased over the last 2 decades. Recent estimates have suggested that 20% of ACL reconstructions are now performed using allograft sources.[2,67]

The impetus for the interest in allograft tissue in ACL reconstructions is primarily due to the morbidity resulting from autograft tissue harvesting. For BPTB grafts, complications include anterior knee pain, patellar tendonitis, patellar rupture, patellar fracture, arthrofibrosis, and quadriceps weakness. Hamstring autografts have been associated with knee flexion weakness, inconsistent graft size, delayed graft-tunnel healing, and fixation difficulties.[45,48,59,68–71] Allografts eliminate donor-site issues, decrease operative time, decrease postoperative pain, improve cosmesis, and allow for larger graft sizes.[1,36–38,57,60]

Though allografts possess their own disadvantages, with increased use and knowledge, many of the original drawbacks have been overcome. Modern tissue banking techniques such as NAT have improved the screening and safety of donor tissues and made disease transmission rare.[72] Traditional sterilization processes using high-dose radiation and ethylene oxide, which have been attributed to early graft failure, have been abandoned for newer graft-friendly techniques such as low-dose radiation and chemical washes.[48] Rehabilitation programs are being modified to accommodate the slower incorporation and maturation time of allografts while still obtaining excellent clinical outcomes.[62] Though progress has been made, modern techniques have yet to completely eliminate the risk of disease transmission, and issues such as immunogenic rejection and delayed biologic incorporation continue to challenge the surgeon.

With the proper indications, allograft tissues in ACL reconstructions can provide the surgeon with results equal to those of autograft reconstructions. As they eliminate donor-site morbidity and decrease surgical time, their use will likely continue to increase in the future. The knowledge and skills to perform a successful allograft ACL reconstruction are essential to any surgeon who operates on the ligamentous structures of the knee.

REFERENCES

1. Guelich DR, Lowe WR, Wilson B. The routine culture of allograft tissue in anterior cruciate ligament reconstruction. Am J Sports Med 2007;35:1495–9.

2. Cohen SB, Sekiya JK. Allograft safety in anterior cruciate ligament reconstruction. Clin Sports Med 2007;26:597–605.
3. Centers for Disease Control and Prevention. About tissue transplants. Available at: http://www.cdc.gov/ncidod/dhqp/tissueTransplantsFAQ.html; 2006. Accessed July 12, 2008.
4. Suarez LS, Richmond JC. Overview of procurement, processing, and sterilization of soft tissue allografts for sports medicine. Knee Surg Sports Traumatol Arthrosc 2003;11:219–22.
5. McAllister DR, Joyce MJ, Barton JM, et al. Allograft update: the current status of tissue regulation, procurement, processing, and sterilization. Am J Sports Med 2007;35:2148–58.
6. Curran AR, Adams DJ, Gill JL, et al. The biomechanical effects of low-dose irradiation on bone-patellar tendon-bone allografts. Am J Sports Med 2004;32:1131–5.
7. Rappe M, Horodyski M, Meister K, et al. Nonirradiated versus irradiated Achilles allograft: in vivo failure comparison. Am J Sports Med 2007;35:1653–8.
8. Cooper DE, Arnoczky SP, Warren RF. Contaminated patellar tendon grafts: incidence of positive cultures and efficacy of an antibiotic solution soak—an in vitro study. Arthroscopy 1991;7:272–4.
9. Molina ME, Nonweiller DE, Evans JA, et al. Contaminated anterior cruciate ligament grafts: the efficacy of 3 sterilization agents. Arthroscopy 2000;16:373–8.
10. Roberts TS, Drez D Jr, McCarthy W, et al. Anterior cruciate ligament reconstruction using freeze-dried, ethylene oxide sterilized, bone-patellar tendon-bone allografts. Two year results in thirty-six patients. Am J Sports Med 1991;19:35–41.
11. Schwartz HE, Matava MJ, Proch FS, et al. The effect of gamma irradiation on anterior cruciate ligament allograft biomechanical and biochemical properties in the caprine model at time zero and at 6 months after surgery. Am J Sports Med 2006;34:1747–55.
12. Silvaggio VJ, Fu FH, Georgescu HI, et al. The induction of IL-1 by freeze-dried ethylene oxide-treated bone-patellar tendon-bone allograft wear particles: an in vitro study. Arthroscopy 1993;9:82–6.
13. Scheffler SU, Gonnermann J, Kamp J, et al. Remodeling of ACL allografts is inhibited by peracetic acid sterilization symposium: new approaches to allograft transplantation. CORR 2008;466(8):1810–8.
14. Belkoff S, Haut R. Microstructurally based model analysis of gamma-irradiated tendon allografts. J Orthop Res 1992;10:461–4.
15. De Deyne P, Haut R. Some effects of gamma irradiation on patellar tendon allografts. Connect Tissue Res 1991;27:51–62.
16. Fideler BM, Vangsness CT Jr, Lu B, et al. Gamma irradiation: effects on biomechanical properties of human bone-patellar tendon-bone allografts. Am J Sports Med 1995;23:643–6.
17. Gibbons M, Butler D, Grood E, et al. Effects of gamma irradiation on the initial mechanical and material properties of goat bone-patellar tendon-bone allografts. J Orthop Res 1991;9:209–18.
18. Salehpour A, Butler DL, Proch FS, et al. Dose-dependent response of gamma irradiation on mechanical properties and related biochemical composition of goat bone-patellar tendon-bone allografts. J Orthop Res 1995;13:898–906.
19. Tomford WW. Transmission of disease through transplantation of musculoskeletal allografts. J Bone Joint Surg Am 1995;77:1742–54.
20. Centers for Disease Control and Prevention (CDC). Hepatitis C virus transmission from an antibody-negative organ and tissue donor—United States, 2000–2002. MMWR Morb Mortal Wkly Rep 2003;52(13):273–6.

21. Barber FA, McGuire DA, Johnson DH. Should allografts be used for routine anterior cruciate ligament reconstructions? Arthroscopy 2003;19:421–5.
22. Buck B, Malinin T, Brown M. Bone transplantation and human immunodeficiency virus: an estimate of risk of acquired immunodeficiency syndrome (AIDS). Clin Orthop Relat Res 1989;240:129–36.
23. Buck BE, Resnick L, Shah SM, et al. Human immunodeficiency virus cultured from bone. Implications for transplantation. Clin Orthop Relat Res 1990;251:249–53.
24. Stevenson S, Arnoczky SP. Transplantation of musculoskeletal tissues. In: Simon SR, editor. Orthopaedic basic science: biology and biomechanics of the musculoskeletal system. Rosemont (IL): AAOS; 2000. p. 567–79.
25. Conrad EU, Gretch DR, Obermeyer KR, et al. Transmission of the hepatitis-C virus by tissue transplantation. J Bone Joint Surg Am 1995;77:214–44.
26. Li CM, Ho YR, Liu YC. Transmission of human immunodeficiency virus through bone transplantation: a case report. J Formos Med Assoc 2001;100:350–1.
27. National Center for Health Statistics. Deaths: final data for 2005. Available at: http://www.cdc.gov/nchs/data/nvsr/nvsr56/nvsr56_10.pdf. Accessed July 12, 2008.
28. Indelli PF, Dillingham M, Fanton G, et al. Septic arthritis in postoperative anterior cruciate ligament reconstruction. Clin Orthop Relat Res 2002;398:182–8.
29. Centers for Disease Control and Prevention. Septic arthritis following anterior cruciate ligament reconstruction using tendon allografts—Florida and Louisiana. MMWR Morb Mortal Wkly Rep 2001;50:1081–3.
30. Centers for Disease Control and Prevention. Unexplained deaths following knee surgery—Minnesota, November 2001. MMWR Morb Mortal Wkly Rep 2001; 50(46):1035–6.
31. Centers for Disease Control and Prevention. Update: allograft-associated bacterial infections—United States, 2002. MMWR Morb Mortal Wkly Rep 2002;51: 207–10.
32. Kainer MA, Linden JV, Whaley DN, et al. Clostridium infections associated with musculoskeletal-tissue allografts. N Engl J Med 2004;350:2564–71.
33. Patel R, Trampuz A. Infections transmitted through musculoskeletal tissue allografts. N Engl J Med 2004;350:2544–6.
34. Centers for Disease Control and Prevention. Invasive Streptococcus pyogenes after allograft implantation—Colorado, 2003. MMWR Morb Mortal Wkly Rep 2003;52:273–4.
35. Diaz-de-Rada P, Barriga A, Barroso JL, et al. Positive culture in allograft ACL-reconstruction: what to do? Knee Surg Sports Traumatol Arthrosc 2003;11: 219–22.
36. Olson EJ. Use of soft tissue allografts in sports medicine. Advances in Operative Orthopaedics 1993;1:111–28.
37. Prodromos CC, Fu FH, Howell SM, et al. Controversies in soft-tissue anterior cruciate ligament reconstruction: grafts, bundles, tunnels, fixation, and harvest. J Am Acad Orthop Surg 2008;16:376–84.
38. Miller MD, Harner CD. The use of allograft: techniques and results. Clin Sports Med 1993;12:757–70.
39. Prodromos CC, Joyce BT, Shi K, et al. A meta-analysis of stability of autografts compared to allografts after anterior cruciate ligament reconstruction. Knee Surg Sports Traumatol Arthrosc 2007;15:851–6.
40. Chang SKY, Egami DK, Shaib MD, et al. Anterior cruciate ligament reconstruction: allograft versus autograft. Arthroscopy 2003;19:453–62.
41. Olson EJ, Fu FH, Irrgang JJ, et al. Anterior cruciate ligament reconstruction with sterilely harvested, fresh frozen allograft: four year results. Presented at the 11th

annual meeting of the Arthroscopy Association of North America. Boston, MA, 1992.
42. Malinin T, Levitt RL, Mnaymneh W, et al. Study of retrieved whole ACL replacement allografts five years post implantation. Presented at the 19th annual meeting of the Arthroscopy Association of North America. Miami Beach, FL, April 2000.
43. Cole DW, Ginn TA, Chen GJ, et al. Cost comparison of anterior cruciate ligament reconstruction: autograft versus allograft. Arthroscopy 2005;21(7):786–90.
44. Falconiero RP, DiStefano VJ, Cook TM. Revascularization and ligamentization of autogenous anterior cruciate ligament grafts in humans. Arthroscopy 1998;14:197–205.
45. Rodeo SA, Arnoczky SP, Torzilli PA, et al. Tendon-healing in a bone tunnel: a biomechanical and histological study in the dog. J Bone Joint Surg Am 1993;75:1795–803.
46. Jackson DW, Grood ES, Goldstein JD, et al. A comparison of patellar tendon autograft and allograft used for anterior cruciate ligament reconstruction in the goat model. Am J Sports Med 1993;21:176–85.
47. Gulotta LV, Rodeo SA. Biology of autograft and allograft healing in anterior cruciate ligament reconstruction. Clin Sports Med 2007;26:509–24.
48. West RV, Harner CD. Graft selection in anterior cruciate ligament reconstruction. Journal of the American Academy of Orthopaedic Surgeons 2005;13:197–207.
49. Harris NL, Indelicato PA, Bloomberg MS, et al. Radiographic and histologic analysis of the tibial tunnel after allograft anterior cruciate ligament reconstruction in goats. Am J Sports Med 2002;30:368.
50. Arnoczky SP, Warren RF, Ashlock MA. Replacement of the anterior cruciate ligament using a patellar tendon allograft. An experimental study. J Bone Joint Surg Am 1986;68:376–85.
51. Shino K, Inoue M, Horibe S, et al. Maturation of allograft tendons transplanted into the knee. An arthroscopic and histological study. J Bone Joint Surg Br 1988;70:556–60.
52. Shino K, Kawasaki T, Hirose H, et al. Replacement of the anterior cruciate ligament by an allogeneic tendon graft. An experimental study in the dog. J Bone Joint Surg Br 1984;66:672–81.
53. Nikolaou PK, Seaber AV, Glisson RR, et al. Anterior cruciate ligament allograft transplantation: long-term function, histology, revascularization, and operative technique. Am J Sports Med 1986;14:348.
54. Malinin TI, Levitt RL, Bashore C, et al. A study of retrieved allografts used to replace anterior cruciate ligaments. Arthroscopy 2002;18(2):163–70.
55. Lee CA, Meyer JV, Shilt JS, et al. Allograft maturation in anterior cruciate ligament reconstruction. Arthroscopy 2004;20(6):46–9.
56. Scheffler SU, Schmidt T, Gangey I, et al. Fresh-frozen free-tendon allografts versus autografts in anterior cruciate ligament reconstruction: delayed remodeling and inferior mechanical function during long-term healing in sheep. Arthroscopy 2008;24(4):448–58.
57. Pearsall AW, Hollis JM, Russell GV, et al. A biomechanical comparison of three lower extremity tendons for ligamentous reconstruction about the knee. Arthroscopy 2003;19:1091–6.
58. Singhal MC, Gardiner JR, Johnson DL. Failure of primary anterior cruciate ligament surgery using anterior tibialis allograft. Arthroscopy 2007;23:469–75.
59. Zhang C, Fan H, Xu H, et al. Histological comparison of the fate of ligamentous insertion after reconstruction of anterior cruciate ligament: autograft vs. allograft. Chin J Traumatol 2006;9:72–6.

60. Noyes FR, Barer-Westin SD. Reconstruction of the anterior cruciate ligament with human allograft: comparison of early and later results. J Bone Joint Surg 1996;23:593–6.
61. Nyland J, Caborn D, Rothbauer J, et al. Two-year outcomes following ACL reconstruction with allograft tibialis anterior tendons: a retrospective study. Knee Surg Sports Traumatol Arthrosc 2003;11:212–8.
62. Nakata K, Shino K, Horibe S, et al. Arthroscopic anterior cruciate ligament reconstruction using fresh-frozen bone plug–free allogeneic tendons: 10-year follow-up. Arthroscopy 2008;24:285–91.
63. Sterling JC, Meyers MC, Calvo RD. Allograft failure in cruciate ligament reconstruction. Follow-up evaluation of eighteen patients. Am J Sports Med 1995;23:173–8.
64. Harner C, Olson E, Irrgang J, et al. Allograft versus autograft anterior cruciate ligament reconstruction: 3–5-year outcome. Clin Orthop 1996;324:134–44.
65. Peterson RK, Shelton WR, Bomboy AL. Allograft versus autograft patellar tendon anterior cruciate ligament reconstruction: a 5-year follow-up. Arthroscopy 2001;17:9–13.
66. Stringham DR, Pelmas CJ, Burks RT, et al. Comparison of anterior cruciate ligament reconstructions using patellar tendon autograft or allograft. Arthroscopy 1996;12:414–21.
67. The American Orthopaedic Society for Sports Medicine Conference on Allografts in Orthopaedic Sports Medicine. Keystone (CO) July 14–17, 2005.
68. Aglietti P, Buzzi R, D'Andria S, et al. Patellofemoral problems after intraarticular anterior cruciate ligament reconstruction. Clin Orthop Relat Res 1993;288:195–204.
69. Sachs RA, Daniel DM, Stone ML, et al. Patellofemoral problems after anterior cruciate ligament reconstruction. Am J Sports Med 1989;17:760–5.
70. Yasuda K, Tsujino J, Ohkoshi Y, et al. Graft site morbidity with autogenous semitendinosus and gracilis tendons. Am J Sports Med 1995;23:706–14.
71. Tuman JM, Diduch DR, Rubino LJ, et al. Predictors for hamstring graft diameter in anterior cruciate ligament reconstruction. Am J Sports Med 2007;35:1945–9.
72. Vangsness C Jr, Wagner P, Moore T, et al. Overview of safety issues concerning the preparation and processing of soft-tissue allografts. Arthroscopy 2006;22:1351–8.

Posterior Cruciate Ligament Reconstruction: Achilles Tendon Allograft, Double Bundle

Andrew D. Heinzelmann, MD, Gene R. Barrett, MD*

KEYWORDS

• Posterior cruciate ligament • Allograft • Achilles tendon

Posterior cruciate ligament (PCL) injuries have historically been underdiagnosed because they are often asymptomatic. However, it now appears that PCL injuries may comprise one-fifth or more of all knee ligament injuries.[1] There is considerable variability in the reported incidence of PCL injury with a review of the literature (in 1999) showing PCL injuries to comprise 1% to 44% of all acute knee injuries.[2] Reports have found PCL injuries to be present in 3% of the general population,[3] and a 2% incidence of asymptomatic, isolated PCL tears was shown in elite college football players.[4] The majority of isolated PCL injuries occur during contact athletics where a posterior force is directed to the proximal tibia of a flexed knee. In trauma patients, it has been reported that 37% of knee injuries involve the PCL and greater than 90% are multi-ligamentous injuries.[5] Despite an increase in diagnosis, the number of PCL reconstructions performed annually is far fewer, and outcomes are less favorable, than with anterior cruciate ligament (ACL) reconstructions.[6] However, with the advent of new technology and techniques, PCL reconstruction is becoming more reproducible and successful.

There are many controversies surrounding PCL reconstruction, including indications, graft choice, allograft verse autograft tissue, and reconstruction technique. In recent years, allografts have become a popular choice in orthopedic sports medicine because they decrease surgical time and morbidity while improving cosmesis and allowing for faster rehabilitation. McAllister and colleagues[7] recently reported that 60,000 allografts were used in knee surgeries by American Orthopaedic Society for

Mississippi Sports Medicine and Orthopaedic Center, Jackson, MS, USA
* Corresponding author.
E-mail address: gbarrett@msmoc.com (G.R. Barrett).

Clin Sports Med 28 (2009) 245–257
doi:10.1016/j.csm.2008.10.013
0278-5919/08/$ – see front matter © 2009 Elsevier Inc. All rights reserved.

Sports Medicine members in 2005. It is estimated that nearly 20% of ACL reconstructions in the United States are completed using allografts,[8] and many orthopedic surgeons prefer allografts for PCL reconstruction. However, allografts are expensive, limited in supply, and carry the inherent risk of disease transmission, immune reaction, and slow incorporation into host tissue. In this article, the indications for PCL reconstruction, graft and technique choices, and allograft safety are discussed and the technique for allograft PCL reconstruction is described.

INDICATIONS FOR PCL RECONSTRUCTION

The most important step in determining an appropriate management strategy is correct diagnosis. The pattern of injury can be acute or chronic, isolated or combined with other ligamentous disruptions. Many isolated PCL disruptions are difficult to diagnose because they are often asymptomatic and comprise a smaller percentage of ligament injuries in the general population than PCL injuries found in the setting of combined ligamentous disruptions.[9-11] To assist in diagnosis, several clinical tests have been described. The posterior drawer test is performed with the patient supine and the knee flexed to 90°. After determining the anterior tibial starting point, a posteriorly directed force is applied to the tibia with the leg in internal, external, and neutral rotation. The test is graded by measuring the distance the anterior tibia translates posteriorly in relation to the distal femur and then compared with the contralateral knee (**Fig. 1**). Posterior tibial translation is 0–5 mm for grade 1, 5–10 mm for grade 2, and >10 mm for grade 3 injuries. The dial or external rotation test is done with the patient prone and the tibia externally rotated at both 30° and 90°. Asymmetry of 15° at 30° of flexion represents an isolated posterolateral corner (PLC) injury; however, asymmetry at both 30° and 90° represents a combined PCL and PLC injury.[12] Posterior stress radiographs are useful to confirm clinical suspicion of a PCL tear and to evaluate graft integrity postoperatively. With the knee flexed to 90°, a posterior force is applied to the proximal tibia, and the amount of posterior tibial translation is quantified and compared with that of the contralateral knee (**Fig. 2**).

It has been shown that a ruptured PCL results in abnormal knee biomechanics, with subsequent degenerative changes in the patellofemoral joint and medial compartment of the knee.[13-16] However, there is conflicting evidence with regard to patient outcome after conservative management for isolated PCL tears. Reports have shown that patients have persistent anterior and medial knee pain, instability, patellofemoral symptoms, and medial compartment degeneration after nonoperative management for isolated PCL injuries.[1,12] In contrast, another study demonstrates that 80% of patients were satisfied with their outcome following nonoperative treatment for isolated

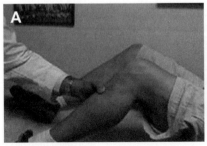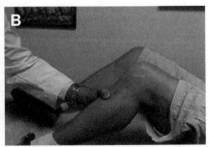

Fig. 1. Posterior drawer test (*A*) before and (*B*) after a posterior force on the proximal tibia.

A   **B**

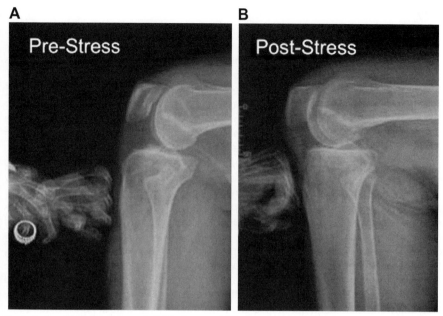

Pre-Stress   Post-Stress

Fig. 2. Lateral tibial radiograph (*A*) before and (*B*) after posterior force on the proximal tibia.

PCL tears and many returned to previous activities.[4] As a result there are many treatment options described for the treatment of acute isolated PCL injuries including nonoperative[4,17–19] and operative[20–23] methods.

Acute isolated grade 1 or 2 injuries are commonly treated with immobilization in extension for 2–4 weeks followed by rehabilitation focusing on normal knee motion and quadriceps strengthening. Shelbourne and Muthukaruppan[24] showed that isolated PCL tears less than grade 3 treated with nonoperative measures showed no deterioration in subjective knee scores at an average of 8.8 years after injury. Treatment of acute grade 3 PCL tears is more controversial. Traditionally, these injuries were treated conservatively with periodic follow-up to assess the development of symptoms or arthrosis; however, most authors now recommend surgical reconstruction for acute isolated grade 3 injuries.[1,25] Asymptomatic patients with chronic PCL injuries are treated with conservative methods; however, if pain or instability develops, then surgical reconstruction may be considered.[12,25] In the setting of a PCL rupture combined with other ligament tears, such as the ACL, medial collateral ligament, or posterolateral complex, knee function is compromised[18,20,22,26,27] and many surgical options exist. Specifically, in combined PCL/PLC injury, most authors advise early repair of both structures.[19,28–30]

SURGICAL TECHNIQUES

Reconstruction of the PCL using a hamstring graft through an open technique was first described by Hey Groves[31] in 1917. Since then methods of reconstruction have advanced to include open and arthroscopic techniques using tibial inlay or transtibial methods with single or double bundles with a variety of graft options. The current literature does not indicate a superior method of fixation, but each method has its own inherent advantages and disadvantages.

Transtibial Technique

Transtibial techniques are performed arthroscopically using standard portals with the addition of a posterior portal for visualization and instrumentation at the tibial attachment of the PCL. The tibial footprint of the PCL is located between the posterior horns of the medial and lateral menisci distal to the tibial plateau in the posterior intercondylar fossa in 2 distinct bundles, anterolateral (AL) and posteromedial (PM) (**Fig. 3**).[32–37] The transtibial technique has the advantage of avoiding a formal posterior approach to the back of the knee, which most surgeons are unfamiliar with, and poses a risk in the revision situation secondary to scar formation adjacent to neurovascular structures.[12] However, the transtibial technique has several difficulties. It is a technically demanding procedure to perform and should be reserved for the experienced knee surgeon who is comfortable with establishing a posterior portal, maintaining visualization, and safely using instruments near neurovascular structures. Fluid extravasation into the posterior compartment of the leg can place the patient at risk for a compartment syndrome. Also, the sharp angle or "killer turn" the graft must make as it comes from the tibial tunnel into the knee joint can potentially make graft passage difficult, increase stress on the graft, and damage the graft by impingement on the roof of the tunnel (**Fig. 4**). Modifications in technique are used to minimize the acute angle the tibial tunnel presents, and a recent cadaveric study[38] found that an AL starting position for the tibial tunnel reduced graft angulation around the posterior aspect of the tibia. Another difficulty the transtibial technique poses is the need for a long graft to achieve adequate fixation in the tunnel. This can limit options for graft choice, especially if bone-patellar tendon-bone (BPTB) grafts are used.

The technique is performed with the patient in the supine position, and standard arthroscopy portals are established. The arthroscope is driven from the AL portal through the notch to the PM compartment to view the tibial attachment of the PCL. A spinal needle is used to localize PM portal placement. Through the PM portal, the PCL footprint is

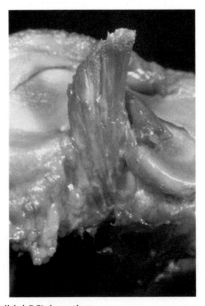

Fig. 3. Posterior view of tibial PCL insertion.

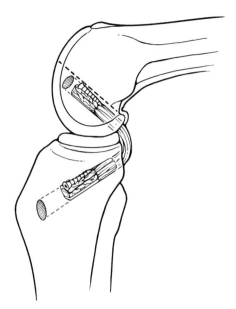

Fig. 4. The "killer turn" created from a transtibial tunnel.

abraded and cleared of soft tissue. Viewing is switched to the anteromedial (AM) portal, and a PCL guide is placed through the AL portal to the insertion site down the back of the tibia. A guide pin is inserted just superior to the pes anserine and visualized as it pierces the posterior cortex. The tunnel is reamed and measured appropriately for the size of graft used. The femoral tunnel can be drilled from outside in or inside out.

Tibial Inlay Technique

Tibial inlay techniques described by Berg[39] were developed to address some of the difficulties inherent to the transtibial technique. Inlay techniques allow direct visualization for tibial preparation and fixation and eliminate the need for graft passage around the "killer turn" created in transtibial techniques. Because the graft is fixed directly onto the posterior tibia, graft length is preserved. Therefore, shorter grafts like BPTB can be used without the risk of graft-tunnel length mismatch. Disadvantages include difficult patient positioning, nonunion of the bone plug to the tibia, unfamiliar approach, and scar formation, which can make revision surgery difficult and dangerous.[12]

Patients are positioned in the lateral decubitus position, and an arthroscopic preparation of the femoral tunnel is completed. A horizontal incision in the knee flexion crease is created. The medial gastrocnemius head is retracted laterally with the neurovascular structures, exposing the posterior capsule. A vertical incision is made in the capsule, and the PCL insertion is visualized and prepared. A unicortical window to match the bone plug is made in the posterior tibial plateau within the tibial anatomic footprint. The bone plug is fixed with screws and washers, and femoral fixation is completed according to the surgeon's preference.[12]

Single Bundle Versus Double Bundle

Both techniques are usually performed arthroscopically. Current single-bundle techniques are designed to replace the stronger AL bundle, which is located more anteriorly on the femur. The tunnel can be drilled in an inside-out or outside-in fashion. The tip of a drill guide is inserted through the AM portal and placed 8 to 9 mm above the articular surface on the anterior half of the PCL footprint. The knee is flexed 70°–90°, and the guide pin is drilled from a position between the medial epicondyle and patella on the outside of the knee. A tunnel is then created by drilling over the wire from inside out[12] or outside in.

Double-bundle techniques have gained popularity because it has been demonstrated that reconstruction of both the AL and PM bundle creates a more anatomic reconstruction and load distribution than single-bundle techniques. Studies have indicated that both bundles are critical to the overall stability of the PCL.[40] The addition of a PM bundle decreases posterior laxity and provides improved stability through full knee range of motion.[41] The technique involves adding a second tunnel more posteriorly over the native PM footprint. Using a single bone block on the tibial side, the 2 graft limbs are passed retrograde and tensioned at 90° of flexion and full extension for the AL and PM bundles, respectively.

Graft Choices

There are many graft options for PCL reconstruction. Graft selection depends on surgeon preference and tissue availability. Ideal grafts have rapid incorporation, good strength and stiffness, and low morbidity.

Autografts

Autologous graft options include BPTB, quadriceps, and hamstring. The bone plugs on the BPTB graft and quadriceps graft provide excellent rigid bony fixation for both transtibial and inlay techniques. However, anterior knee pain, especially with BPTB autografts, and graft-tunnel mismatch can occur. Graft length can be problematic when using transtibial techniques, and some autografts may be too short for optimal fixation.

Allografts

There are many allograft options available including Achilles tendon, BPTB, quadriceps, and soft tissue grafts such as hamstring and tibialis anterior or posterior tendons. Allograft tissue is often preferred in PCL reconstruction because of the advantages in avoiding graft-tunnel mismatch, decreasing surgical time and donor-site morbidity,[13,42,43] as well as improving cosmesis. Allografts are very useful in combined injuries in which autograft tissue can be limited and multiple reconstructions may be necessary. Disadvantages of allograft tissue include high cost, limited availability, risk of disease transmission, slowed graft incorporation, tissue rejection, and alteration of the graft's structural properties by sterilization and storage procedures.[26,44,45] Previous reports have shown disease transmission from allograft tissue.[7,46,47] These risks should be discussed with the patient before proceeding with an allograft.

Of the allografts available, we prefer the Achilles tendon for PCL reconstruction for a variety of reasons. There have been many reports of successful PCL reconstruction using Achilles tendon allograft tissue.[48–56] Also, Achilles tendon grafts have a large bone plug that can be fashioned to an appropriate size for both transtibial and inlay techniques. In addition, there is abundant tendon length and thickness for both single-bundle and double-bundle reconstruction techniques (**Fig. 5**), which avoids graft-tunnel length mismatch. The inherent disadvantages of Achilles allograft are true of all allografts and include risk of disease transmission, limited availability, and high cost.

Author's (G.R.B.) Preferred Technique

An Achilles tendon allograft through a transtibial tunnel with double-bundle femoral fixation is preferred.

Graft preparation

A fresh-frozen Achilles allograft tendon from a reputable firm is thawed in a room temperature, normal saline, antibiotic solution for 15 minutes before starting the surgical procedure. The distal bony calcaneal attachment of the graft is typically fashioned to a 25 × 11 mm bone block. One 2.5-mm hole is drilled through the center of the bone plug. A No. 5 braided nonabsorbable suture is passed through the drill hole. A second No. 5 braided nonabsorbable suture is also passed through the drill hole and then back through the tendon-bone interface and back through the bone plug in a figure-of-eight fashion. The tendinous portion of the graft is split in line with the fibers, creating 2 tails, one 7 mm and one 9 mm, and cut to produce a total graft length of 15 cm (**Fig. 5**). The graft is placed onto a graft preparation and tensioning board, and a No. 5 braided nonabsorbable suture is placed in a whipstitch fashion into both tails of the tendinous portion of the graft. The graft is tensioned at 20 lb for 15 minutes while being covered with an antibiotic-solution-soaked gauze.

Diagnostic arthroscopy

Superolateral outflow, AM, and AL viewing portals are established. A diagnostic arthroscopy is performed, and concomitant meniscal or chondral injury is addressed. A PM portal is established using a 70° arthroscope, and the tibial attachment of the PCL is identified and decorticated with care to protect the surrounding neurovascular structures. An angled curette can be used to start this process, and a curved mechanical shaver can complete it.

PCL reconstruction

Viewing from the PM portal, a PCL drill guide is placed through the AM portal onto the decorticated PCL footprint. A small incision is made on the AM tibial flare, and a guide pin is advanced through the tibia under fluoroscopic C-arm control (**Fig. 6**). Placement should be just anterior to the posterior tibial corner. The tunnel is reamed progressively larger from an 8-mm reamer to an 11-mm reamer with the posterior cortex reamed by hand to avoid neurovascular injury. The anterior edge of the tunnel is smoothed with a curette. To avoid the "killer turn," this pin should be at a gentle angle just anterior to the posterior tibial corner.

A small incision is made over the vastus medialis obliquus (VMO), and it is retracted anteriorly. The femoral attachment of the PCL is visualized. The anatomic footprint of the AL femoral bundle is found approximately 7 mm from the articular cartilage in the 10:30 position for a left knee and 1:30 position for a right knee,[33] and the anatomic footprint of the PM femoral bundle is found 4–5 mm posterior to the articular junction

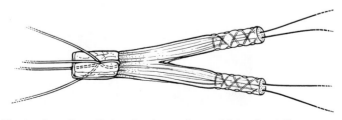

Fig. 5. Achilles tendon allograft showing bone plug and 2 tendon tails.

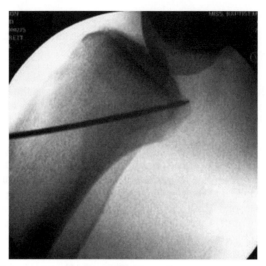

Fig. 6. Guide pin placement for the transtibial tunnel.

in the 3 o'clock position for a right knee and the 9 o'clock position for a left knee (**Fig. 7**). A femoral guide is placed on the femoral footprint of the AL bundle through the AM portal. A guide pin is advanced from outside in, and a 9-mm tunnel is reamed. Then, the drill guide is placed on the femoral footprint of the PM bundle, and a 7-mm tunnel is reamed.

The graft is passed through the tibial tunnel so that the bone plug remains in the tibial tunnel and the 2 tendinous tails are brought into the knee. An interference screw is advanced from anterior to posterior over a guidewire into the tibial tunnel to lock the bone plug in place. First the 7-mm allograft bundle is passed into the PM tunnel followed by the 9-mm allograft bundle into the AL tunnel. The knee is placed in 0° to 5° of extension and an 8- to 9-mm absorbable interference screw is advanced into the PM femoral tunnel over a guidewire from outside in. Lastly, the knee is flexed to 90°, and a 10-mm absorbable interference screw is advanced into the AL tunnel over a guidewire from

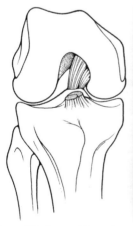
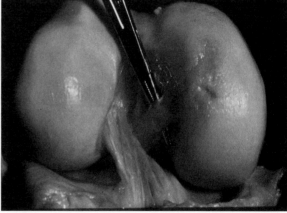

Fig. 7. PCL femoral insertion.

outside in, with an anteriorly directed force applied to the proximal tibia. The graft is visualized (**Fig. 8**) and taken through a gentle range of motion. Posterior and posterolateral drawer tests are done to confirm adequate fixation and stability.

Wound closure
The wounds are irrigated with Betadine (povidon iodine) solution and antibiotic irrigant, and hemostasis is obtained. An absorbable 2-0 braided suture is used for subcutaneous closure, and a 0 nonabsorbable monofilament suture is used in a running fashion in the subcuticular layer; then Steri-Strips adhesive skin closures are applied. The skin is infiltrated with local anesthetic, a drain is placed through the superomedial outflow portal, and the remaining portals are closed. Betadine-soaked nonadherent gauze and 4 × 4s cover the wounds, and a sterile bandage and knee immobilizer are applied. Dorsalis pedis and posterior tibialis pulses are identified immediately after surgery. Patients are admitted to 23-hour observation for cryotherapy, drain management, and pain control. The drain is discontinued on postoperative day 1, and the dressing is changed.

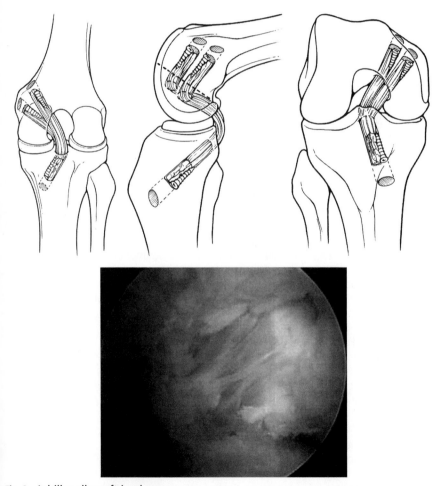

Fig. 8. Achilles allograft in place.

Rehabilitation Protocol

PCL rehabilitation is progressed more slowly than most accelerated ACL rehabilitation protocols. It is important to allow initial ligament healing to occur before stressing the graft with range-of-motion exercises.[57] We prefer the following rehabilitation protocol. The patient is in a knee brace locked in full extension for the first 2 weeks. Patients are non-weight bearing with 2 crutches for the first 4 weeks. From weeks 2 to 4, passive range of motion in a hinged postoperative brace is allowed from 10° to 90°. At postoperative week 4, motion is allowed from 10° to 120° in the brace. Quadriceps strengthening is started at postoperative week 3 and continued throughout the entire rehabilitation process with specific avoidance of hamstring strengthening until 3 months after surgery. At 3 months postoperatively, the brace is discontinued, and patients should have symmetric motion with a normal gait pattern. From 3 to 6 months, hamstring strengthening is started, and the patient is allowed to jog in a brace. Return to sports and heavy labor is allowed 9 months postoperatively when strength, range of motion, and proprioceptive skills are symmetric to the uninjured side.

SUMMARY

There are many accepted graft and technique choices available for reconstruction of the PCL. The use of allograft tissue has been shown to be a successful and reproducible procedure. The advantages of using allograft tissue are decreased operative time, decreased surgical morbidity, and improved cosmesis and graft versatility for both primary and revision cases. However, there is still concern about tissue safety, cost, graft incorporation, and graft rejection. It is important for surgeons to discuss the risks and benefits of allograft tissue with their patients before proceeding with allograft reconstruction.

REFERENCES

1. Cosgarea AJ, Jay PR. Posterior cruciate ligament injuries: evaluation and management. J Am Acad Orthop Surg 2001;9:297–307.
2. Shelbourne KD, Davis TJ, Patel DV. The natural history of acute, isolated, nonoperatively treated posterior cruciate ligament injuries: a prospective study. Am J Sports Med 1999;27:276–83.
3. Miyasaka KC, Daniel DM. The incidence of knee ligament injuries in the general population. Am J Knee Surg 1991;4:3–8.
4. Parolie JM, Bergfeld JA. Long-term results of nonoperative treatment of isolated posterior cruciate ligament injuries in the athlete. Am J Sports Med 1986;14:35–8.
5. Fanelli GC, Edson CJ. Posterior cruciate ligament injuries in trauma patients: part II. Arthroscopy 1995;11:526–9.
6. Harner CD, Fu FH, Irrgang JJ, et al. Anterior and posterior cruciate ligament reconstruction in the new millennium: a global perspective. Knee Surg Sports Traumatol Arthrosc 2001;9:330–6.
7. McAllister DR, Joyce MJ, Mann BJ, et al. Allograft update: the current status of tissue regulation, procurement, processing, and sterilization. Am J Sports Med 2007;35:2148–58.
8. Cohen SB, Sekiya JK. Allograft safety in anterior cruciate ligament reconstruction. Clin Sports Med 2007;26:597–605.
9. Trickey EL. Injuries to the posterior cruciate ligament. Clin Orthop 1980;147:76–81.
10. Fanelli GC. PCL injuries in trauma patients. Arthroscopy 1993;9(3):291–4.

11. Bergfeld JA. Diagnosis and non-operative treatment of acute posterior cruciate ligament injury. Instr Course Lect AAOS 1990;208.
12. Battaglia TC, Mulhall KJ, Miller MD. Posterior cruciate ligament. In: Johnson DL, Mair SD, editors. Clinical sports medicine. 1st edition. Philadelphia: Mosby, Elsevier; 2006. p. 547–59.
13. Bullis DW, Paulos LE. Reconstruction of the posterior cruciate ligament with allograft. Clin Sports Med 1994;13:581–97.
14. Clancy WG. Repair and reconstruction of the posterior cruciate ligament. In: Chapman M, editor. Operative orthopaedics. Philadelphia: JB Lippincott; 1988. p. 1651–65.
15. Cross MJ, Powell JF. Long term follow up of posterior cruciate ligament rupture: a study of 116 cases. Am J Sports Med 1984;12:292–7.
16. Gill TJ, DeFrate LE, Wang C, et al. The effect of posterior cruciate ligament reconstruction on patellofemoral contact pressures in the knee joint under simulated muscle loads. Am J Sports Med 2004;32:109–15.
17. Fowler PJ, Messieh SS. Isolated posterior cruciate ligament injuries in athletes. Am J Sports Med 1987;15:553–7.
18. Torg JS, Barton JM. Natural history of the posterior cruciate deficient knee. Clin Orthop 1989;246:208–16.
19. Noyes FR, Barber-Westin SD. Treatment of complex injuries involving the posterior cruciate and posterolateral ligaments of the knee. Am J Knee Surg 1996;9: 200–14.
20. Johnson JC, Bach BR. Current concepts review, posterior cruciate ligament. Am J Knee Surg 1990;3:143–53.
21. Clancy WG Jr, Shelbourne KD, Zoellner GB, et al. Treatment of knee joint instability secondary to rupture of the posterior cruciate ligament: report of a new procedure. J Bone Joint Surg Am 1983;65:310–22.
22. Veltri DM, Warren RF. Isolated and combined posterior cruciate ligament injuries. J Am Acad Orthop Surg 1993;1:67–75.
23. Loss WC, Fox JM, Blazina ME, et al. Acute posterior cruciate ligament injuries. Am J Sports Med 1981;9:86–92.
24. Shelbourne KD, Muthukaruppan Y. Subjective results of nonoperatively treated, acute, isolated posterior cruciate ligament injuries. Arthroscopy 2005;21(4):457–61.
25. Fanelli GC, Giannotti BF, Edson CJ. The posterior cruciate ligament arthroscopic evaluation and treatment. Arthroscopy 1994;10:673–88.
26. Marks PH, Cameron M, Fu FH. Reconstruction of the cruciate ligaments with allogenic transplants: techniques, results and perspectives. Orthopade 1993; 22:386–91.
27. Clancy WG. Knee ligamentous injury in sports: the past, present, and future. Med Sci Sports 1983;15:9–14.
28. Watanabe Y, Moriya H, Takahashi K, et al. Functional anatomy of the posterolateral structures of the knee. Arthroscopy 1993;9:57–62.
29. Hughston JC, Jacobson KE. Chronic posterolateral rotatory instability of the knee. J Bone Joint Surg Am 1985;67:351–9.
30. De Lee JC, Riley MB, Rockwood CA. Acute posterolateral rotatory instability of the knee. Am J Sports Med 1983;11:199–207.
31. Hey Groves EW. Operation for repair of the cruciate ligaments. Lancet 1917;2: 674–5.
32. Amis AA, Gupte CM, Bull AMJ, et al. Anatomy of the posterior cruciate ligament and the meniscofemoral ligaments. Knee Surg Sports Traumatol Arthrosc 2005; 14:257–63.

33. Edwards A, Bull MJ, Amis AA. The attachments of the fiber bundles of the posterior cruciate ligament: an anatomic study. Arthroscopy 2007;23(3):284–90.
34. Harner CD, Baek GH, Vogrin TM, et al. Quantitative analysis of human cruciate ligament insertions. Arthroscopy 1999;15:741–9.
35. Makris CA, Georgoulis AD, Papageorgiou CD, et al. Posterior cruciate ligament architecture: evaluation under microsurgical dissection. Arthroscopy 2000;16:627–32.
36. Morgan CD, Kalman VR, Grawl DM. The anatomic origin of the posterior cruciate ligament: where is it? Reference landmarks for PCL reconstruction. Arthroscopy 1997;13:325–31.
37. Takahashi M, Matsubara T, Doi M, et al. Anatomical study of the femoral and tibial insertions of the anterolateral and posteromedial bundles of human posterior cruciate ligament. Knee Surg Sports Traumatol Arthrosc 2006;14:1055–9.
38. Huang TW, Wang CJ, Weng LH, et al. Reducing the "killer turn" in posterior cruciate ligament reconstruction. Arthroscopy 2003;19:712–6.
39. Berg EE. Posterior cruciate ligament tibial inlay reconstruction. Arthroscopy 1995;11:69–76.
40. Fox RJ, Harner CD, Sakane M, et al. Determination of the in situ forces in the human posterior cruciate ligament using robotic technology: a cadaveric study. Am J Sports Med 1998;26:395–401.
41. Harner CD, Janaushek MA, Kanamori A, et al. Biomechanical analysis of double-bundle posterior cruciate ligament reconstruction. Am J Sports Med 2000;28:144–51.
42. Fanelli GC, Giannotti BF, Edson CJ. Arthroscopically assisted combined posterior cruciate ligament/posterolateral complex reconstruction. Arthroscopy 1996;12:521–30.
43. Noyes FR, Barber-Westin SD. Posterior cruciate ligament allograft reconstruction with and without augmentation device. Arthroscopy 1994;10:317–82.
44. Pinkowski JL, Reiman PR, Chen S. Human lymphocyte reaction to freeze-dried allograft and xenograft ligamentous tissue. Am J Sports Med 1989;17:595–600.
45. Shino K, Oakes BW, Horibe S, et al. Collagen fibril populations in human anterior cruciate ligament allografts: electron microscopic analysis. Am J Sports Med 1995;23:203–9.
46. Asselmeier MA, Caspari RB, Bottenfield RB. A review of allograft processing and sterilization techniques and their role in transmission of the human immunodeficiency virus. Am J Sports Med 1993;21:170–5.
47. Vangsness CT Jr, Garcia IA, Mills CR, et al. Allograft transplantation in the knee: tissue regulation, procurement, processing, and sterilization. Am J Sports Med 2003;31:474–81.
48. Ahn JH, Yoo JC, Wang JH. Posterior cruciate ligament reconstruction: double-loop hamstring tendon autograft versus Achilles tendon allograft—clinical results of a minimum 2-year follow-up. Arthroscopy 2005;21(8):965–9.
49. DeBeradino TM, Lonergan KT, Brooks DE. Comparison of the split stacked versus the split achilles allograft for dual femoral tunnel posterior cruciate ligament reconstruction. Am J Sports Med 2008;36(1):142–8.
50. Dennis MG, Fox JA, Alford JW, et al. Posterior cruciate ligament reconstruction. J Knee Surg 2004;17:133–9.
51. Kim SJ, Park IS. Arthroscopic reconstruction of the posterior cruciate ligament using tibial-inlay and double-bundle technique. Arthroscopy 2005;21(10):1271.e1–6.
52. Mariani PP, Margheritini F. Full arthroscopic inlay reconstruction of posterior cruciate ligament. Knee Surg Sports Traumatol Arthrosc 2006;14:1038–44.

53. Sekiya JK, West RV, Ong BC, et al. Clinical outcomes after isolated arthroscopic single-bundle posterior cruciate ligament reconstruction. Arthroscopy 2005; 21(9):1042–50.
54. Wind WM, Bergfeld JA, Parker RD. Evaluation and treatment of posterior cruciate ligament injuries: revisited. Am J Sports Med 2004;32(7):1765–75.
55. Yoon KH, Bae DK, Song SJ, et al. Arthroscopic double-bundle augmentation of posterior cruciate ligament using split achilles allograft. Arthroscopy 2005; 21(12):1436–42.
56. Fanelli GC, Edson CJ. Combined posterior cruciate ligament-posterolateral reconstructions with Achilles tendon allograft and biceps femoris tendon tenodesis: 2- to 10-year follow-up. Arthroscopy 2004;20(4):339–45.
57. Fanelli GC. Posterior cruciate ligament rehabilitation: how slow should we go? Arthroscopy 2008;24(2):234–5.

Meniscal Allograft Transplantation

Jonathan D. Packer, MD[a], Scott A. Rodeo, MD[a,b],*

KEYWORDS

• Meniscal • Meniscus • Allograft • Transplantation
• Transplant • Replacement

The menisci play an important role in load transmission, shock absorption, stability, and articular cartilage nutrition in the knee joint. The medial meniscus contributes to joint stability,[1,2] whereas the lateral meniscus has a greater role in load transmission during weight bearing.[3–5] These functions are compromised in menisci that are damaged or torn. When meniscal repair is not possible, partial or total meniscectomy is often required. In 1948, Fairbank[6] first described the natural history of post-meniscectomy patients. Meniscus-deficient knees experience increased articular contact pressure[7–10] and typically progress to joint degeneration.[6,11–14] Meniscal allograft transplantation has emerged as a treatment option for selected meniscus-deficient patients to decrease the articular contact stress, provide pain relief, and restore normal knee kinematics.

EVALUATION OF THE PATIENT FOLLOWING MENISCECTOMY

A patient who has undergone prior meniscectomy should be carefully examined for early onset of joint degeneration. The physical examination should focus on the presence of effusion, joint-line tenderness, crepitus, stability, and axial alignment. Patient evaluation should include flexion weight-bearing radiographs, standing hip-to-ankle films, and magnetic resonance imaging (MRI) with high-resolution cartilage pulse-sequences. Long leg radiographs are used to assess axial alignment. MRI is the most sensitive technique for detecting early hyaline cartilage changes. High-resolution MRI with appropriate pulse sequences (proton-density-weighted fast-spin echo) allows evaluation of the amount of remaining meniscus and can detect subchondral marrow edema, subchondral bone remodeling, and early softening and fibrillation of hyaline cartilage.[15] Bone scans[16] can also aid in detection of early arthrosis.

[a] Laboratory for Soft Tissue Research, Hospital for Special Surgery, 535 East 70th Street, New York, NY 10021, USA
[b] Sports Medicine and Shoulder Service, Hospital for Special Surgery, 535 East 70th Street, New York, NY 10021, USA
* Corresponding author. Hospital for Special Surgery, 535 East 70th Street, New York, NY 10021.
E-mail address: rodeos@hss.edu (S.A. Rodeo).

Clin Sports Med 28 (2009) 259–283
doi:10.1016/j.csm.2008.10.011
0278-5919/08/$ – see front matter © 2009 Elsevier Inc. All rights reserved.

sportsmed.theclinics.com

CLINICAL INDICATIONS FOR MENISCUS TRANSPLANTATION

At present, there are 4 specific clinical situations in which meniscus transplantation may be considered. The indications include early articular cartilage damage, meniscus transplantation combined with cartilage resurfacing or osteotomy, anterior cruciate ligament reconstruction with medial meniscus deficiency, and prophylactic transplantation.

Articular Cartilage Damage

A patient with symptoms referable to a meniscus-deficient tibiofemoral compartment is the most common indication for meniscal transplant. Numerous studies have reported poor clinical outcomes for meniscal transplantation in the setting of advanced joint degeneration.[17–20] Therefore, most authors recommend limiting meniscus transplantation to patients with only early hyaline cartilage degeneration (Outerbridge grade I or II).[17,18,20–22] Lesions with erosion to the subchondral bone (Outerbridge grade IV) are generally considered a contraindication to this procedure. It is critical that meniscus transplantation be performed in a stable knee with normal axial alignment (ie, do not transplant a medial meniscus into a varus knee).

The size and location of hyaline cartilage lesions are important factors in evaluating a meniscal transplant candidate, although further information is required. A small lesion may have no deleterious effects on the mechanical environment if the weight-bearing load can be distributed around its periphery by normal surrounding cartilage. It is difficult to grade many lesions due to varying amounts of hyaline cartilage damage on different locations of the articular surfaces. The flexion weight-bearing zone of the posterior femoral or tibial condyles consists of both meniscal and non-meniscal weight-bearing areas.[5] Focal erosive lesions in this region should be carefully evaluated. The lesions can be detected by MRI and flexion weight-bearing radiographs (early joint-space narrowing). The ideal meniscus transplant candidate would be an individual with only small or partial-thickness chondral lesions in the meniscal weight-bearing zone.

Meniscal Transplantation Combined with Chondral Resurfacing Procedures

Loss of cartilage in the meniscal weight-bearing zone predisposes the meniscus transplant to failure. This is the setting in which concomitant cartilage resurfacing may be considered. Meniscus transplants may help protect the healing cartilage surface by decreasing the chondral contact stresses across the involved compartment. A healthier articular surface should also aid in the healing and ultimate survival of a meniscus transplant. Microfracture is recommended for focal chondral defects that are well contained within essentially normal surrounding cartilage and that are less than 10 mm in diameter. The use of osteochondral tissue is preferred for lesions greater than 10 mm in diameter. Autograft tissue is recommended for lesions up to 15 to 20 mm in diameter. Osteochondral allograft (OA) tissue is used for lesions over 20 mm in diameter. Osteochondral tissue has the advantage of providing the lesion with immediate protection. Microfracture or autologous chondrocyte implantation (ACI) requires time for healing and maturation of the surface. Therefore, in these cases a more conservative rehabilitation program is recommended with 8 to 12 weeks of non–weight bearing if combined with meniscus transplantation.

There is currently minimal evidence in the literature in support of combined meniscus transplantation and resurfacing procedures. Several studies[19,23–25] have followed these combined procedures and reported improvements in both clinical outcomes and satisfactory healing of the transplant based on direct evaluation of the meniscus.

When compared with isolated meniscus transplants, no differences were found in clinical improvements, complication rate, the number of re-operations, or the patient's perception of the knee condition.

Articular Cartilage Damage with Axial Malalignment

Axial alignment should be considered in the evaluation of all knees with articular cartilage pathology. Degeneration of 1 compartment may lead to a varus or valgus deformity. Meniscal transplant failure rates are high when transplanted in the setting of axial malalignment.[17,26] The mechanical axes of both limbs can be accurately determined with weight-bearing hip-to-ankle radiographs on a long cassette. In a normal knee, the mechanical axis generally passes through or just medial to the center of the knee (between the tibial spines). The width of the tibial plateau is measured to determine the 50% point (middle of the tibial width). A mechanical axis that passes between 40% and 60% of the tibial width (less than 10% deviation) is accepted (**Fig. 1**).

Meniscal Transplantation Combined with Osteotomy

It has been established that symptomatic arthritis can recur 5 to 10 years after realignment osteotomy.[27] These results are based on long-term follow-up studies on patients who underwent meniscectomy followed by osteotomy. In theory, restoration of the meniscus should be beneficial. The hypothesis that concomitant meniscus transplantation and osteotomy will delay recurrence of symptoms, however, is supported by minimal evidence. There is a lack of long-term studies evaluating whether combining meniscus transplantation with osteotomy will delay joint degeneration as compared with osteotomy alone. Verdonk and colleagues[28] reported the long-term results of

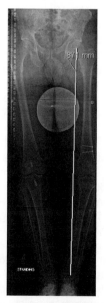

Fig. 1. The mechanical axis should be measured on weight-bearing hip-to-ankle radiographs. A mechanical axis that passes between 40% and 60% of the tibial width is acceptable. In this patient, the mechanical axis passes well medial of the 50% point. A valgus-producing tibial osteotomy was performed before medial meniscal allograft transplantation.

27 medial meniscal transplants (MMTs). The patients who also underwent high tibial osteotomy (HTO) had significantly greater improvements in pain and function scores than those who underwent isolated transplants. In a survivorship analysis, Verdonk and colleagues[29] found that the 10-year survival rates were 83.3% for the group with combined MMT and osteotomy compared with 74.2% for the MMT group without osteotomy. It is unknown, however, whether the clinical improvement can be attributed to the meniscal transplant, the osteotomy, or both.

A malaligned knee may possibly be made suitable for meniscus transplant if corrected by osteotomy. In a varus deformity, a valgus-producing osteotomy should be combined with MMT. Conversely, in a valgus deformity, a varus-producing osteotomy should be combined with lateral meniscus transplantation. Meniscus transplantation with concomitant osteotomy is considered if two conditions are met: (1) there are no architectural changes in the femoral condyle (flattening), and (2) there are no areas of full-thickness cartilage loss greater than 10 mm on the meniscus weight-bearing zone of the femoral or tibial condyles.

Ligament Instability

The medial meniscus has been shown to act as a secondary restraint to anterior tibial translation in the ACL-deficient knee.[1,2] In a cadaveric study, Papageorgiou and colleagues[30] reported significantly increased in situ forces in an ACL graft in medial meniscus–deficient knees compared with meniscus-intact knees. Several studies have provided clinical evidence for the importance of the medial meniscus in knee stability. Shelbourne and Gray[4] demonstrated greater laxity with KT-1000 arthrometer measurements following ACL reconstruction in patients who had undergone previous medial meniscectomy compared with knees with intact menisci. Garrett[18] found that in medial meniscus–deficient patients who underwent ACL reconstructions, the group with concomitant MMT had significantly improved KT-1000 arthrometer results compared with the group with isolated ACL reconstruction. Van Arkel and de Boer[17] also demonstrated improved anterior stability following meniscal transplantation. These data support MMT in ACL reconstruction if the medial meniscus is absent, which is commonly seen during revision ACL reconstruction.

The absence of both the medial and lateral menisci may result in slightly increased varus/valgus rotation,[31] and meniscus transplantation may be considered in this setting if collateral ligament repair or reconstruction is performed. Transplanting both the medial and lateral meniscus may improve varus/valgus stability.

Meniscal Transplantation Combined with ACL Reconstruction

It has been well established that meniscus repairs have superior healing in stable knees.[32,33] As a result, ligament stabilization is recommended either before or concomitantly with meniscus transplantation in an unstable knee. ACL insufficiency is commonly associated with early arthrosis due to previous meniscectomy. Various reconstructive strategies have been reported, including isolated ACL reconstruction,[4,34] isolated osteotomy,[27] or ACL reconstruction combined with osteotomy.[35] Given that there are higher strains in an ACL graft in medial meniscus–deficient knees,[30] concomitant MMT may be considered at the time of ACL reconstruction to help protect the ACL graft. Rueff and colleagues[36] reported a series of 8 ACL reconstructions combined with meniscus transplant that were compared with age-, sex-, and activity-matched patients with ACL reconstruction and either meniscal repair or partial meniscectomy. Both groups displayed similar clinical improvements in modified Lysholm and International Knee Documentation Committee (IKDC) scores, but the transplant group had greater pain improvement.

Early Transplantation

The ultimate goal is to identify meniscal transplant candidates before further articular cartilage degeneration. It is hoped that sophisticated imaging techniques such as MRI will identify these patients while chondral degeneration is still in its early stages. Newer imaging modalities include measurement of T2 relaxation times (a measure of collagen organization), T1 rho (proteoglycan content), MRI, bone scans, and synovial fluid analyses. A difficult decision for the clinician is how early to consider meniscus transplantation. This procedure is not currently recommended for asymptomatic patients with normal articular surfaces. However, meniscus transplant is considered once the asymptomatic patient presents with symptoms and signs of articular cartilage degeneration, such as the development of effusion or changes seen on MRI. The presence of cartilage degeneration indicates increased articular contact stress in the meniscectomized compartment. The contact stresses on articular cartilage increase proportionally with meniscus loss.[7,8]

Portions of the meniscus that are located in the regions of greatest load in weight bearing are thought to provide the most protection to the articular cartilage surface. Li and colleagues[37] found that the point of greatest articular contact stress moved posteriorly with progressive knee flexion in the lateral compartment. Because the posterior horn bears a greater load during knee flexion,[5] its absence likely contributes to a more rapid progression of arthritis. Knowledge of the critical level of stress that initiates progressive cartilage degeneration would help refine indications for meniscus transplant. Unfortunately, this information is not yet available.

The lateral meniscus transmits a greater proportion of load in the lateral compartment during weight bearing than the medial meniscus.[5] As a result, lateral meniscectomy causes more rapid degenerative changes than medial meniscectomy.[11,12] Therefore, meniscus replacement should be considered more aggressively for the lateral meniscus. Lateral meniscus transplantation is currently recommended in patients with greater than 50% removal of the posterior horn. MMT should be considered once 60% to 70% of the posterior horn has been removed.

There are 3 relatively common clinical scenarios that result in meniscal loss in the lateral compartment: (1) The irreparable radial split tear that extends to the capsule. The disruption of circumferential collagen fibers results in loss of hoop stress transmission, which is functionally equivalent to total meniscectomy. (2) The symptomatic discoid lateral meniscus that necessitates subtotal or total meniscectomy. (3) The irreparable bucket-handle tear that involves the majority of the lateral meniscus.

Staging Combined Procedures

Complex knee reconstructions may require meniscus transplant, cartilage resurfacing, ligament reconstruction, and osteotomy. It is often more practical to stage combined procedures due to the magnitude of combined procedures. Osteotomy should be performed before or in conjunction with meniscus transplant and/or cartilage resurfacing. If osteotomy, resurfacing, and meniscus transplant are all desired, then osteotomy is recommended as the first stage followed by meniscus transplant and cartilage resurfacing as a combined second stage.

Contraindications

Absolute contraindications to meniscus transplantation include the presence of diffuse subchondral bone exposure, remodeling of the femoral condyle that has resulted in flattening, and uncorrected malalignment or instability.[19] Due to the poor results in patients with advanced arthritis,[18,20–22,38] meniscus transplantation should be avoided in the presence of a large area of subchondral bone exposure (grade IV lesions) with radiographic joint-space narrowing. However, cartilage damage is often spread out over different parts of the articular surfaces, making it difficult to identify the most problematic lesions.

Progressive degeneration of the posterior portion of the transplanted meniscus is the most common cause of allograft failures. Therefore, full-thickness articular cartilage lesions on the flexion weight-bearing zone that are greater than 10 to 15 mm in width or length should be considered a contraindication.[20] The mechanical axis of the limb should not go through the involved compartment (ie, MMT in a varus knee). Correction of malalignment and/or chondral degeneration with osteotomy and cartilage resurfacing, respectively, may render a knee suitable for meniscus transplantation; however, further studies are necessary to define the indications for such combined procedures.

Changes in bone morphology should also be considered. Studies have reported inferior results with remodeling and flattening of the femoral condyle.[20,22] MRI and radiographs of the knee in full extension and flexion weight-bearing views should be carefully evaluated to detect these morphologic changes.[39]

Graft Type and Processing

Four types of meniscus allografts are currently available. Fresh and cryopreserved allografts contain viable cells, while fresh-frozen and lyophilized allografts are acellular. Fresh grafts have the theoretical advantage of harboring viable cells, but the proportion of cells that survive and the duration of cell survival following transplantation are not known. In a goat model, Jackson and colleagues[40] found that the donor cells in a fresh graft were completely replaced by host cells within 4 weeks. Fresh grafts also introduce several logistical problems, such as transportation, increased disease risk, and operative timing. Cryopreservation has the benefits of maintaining cell membrane integrity and donor fibrochondrocyte viability as well as prolonged storage time. The fate of a cryopreserved graft is unknown, but it is likely that some degree of cellular repopulation with host cells occurs. The importance of viable donor cells remains unclear, which calls into question the advantage of allografts that contain living cells.

Fresh-frozen grafts undergo a freezing process that kills all donor cells and denatures histocompatibility antigens, which may decrease immunogenicity. Fresh-frozen grafts are easier to process and less expensive than cryopreserved grafts. In a goat study, Fabbriciani and colleagues[41] compared cryopreserved and deep-frozen grafts and did not find any advantage of one graft over the other. Lyophilized allografts are not currently recommended because they are susceptible to shrinkage[42] and synovitis[43] and have altered material properties.

Additionally, the allograft may be secondarily sterilized with ethylene oxide, gamma irradiation, or newer proprietary allograft processing techniques. Sterilization should not be performed on fresh or cryopreserved allografts because the process is generally lethal to viable cells. Ethylene oxide is not recommended because one of the by-products (ethylene chlorohydrin) has been found to induce synovitis.[43] Gamma irradiation may be used, but doses required to denature viral DNA (>3.0 Mrad) may have detrimental effects on the material properties of the allograft.[44] The use of fresh-frozen, nonirradiated allografts is currently recommended.

GRAFT SIZING

The biomechanical function of the meniscus transplant relies on proper size matching of the transplant to the recipient knee. Allograft sizing can be determined with either intraoperative or radiographic measurements of the meniscus or tibial plateau. Sizing by intraoperative measurements is not currently recommended, because its accuracy is not known. Previous meniscectomy often precludes direct measurements of the involved meniscus. Therefore, most tissue banks currently size the meniscus based on bone measurements. Studies have demonstrated a consistent relationship between meniscus size and radiographic landmarks.[45–47] However, these studies have also found significant variability in the relationship of meniscal length and width to tibial plateau dimensions. For example, Pollard and colleagues[46] reported measurement error up to 8.4% or 3.8 mm.

Radiographic sizing methods include plain radiographs, MRI, and computed tomography (CT) scans, but controversy exists about which imaging modality is most accurate.[18,48–51] Shaffer and colleagues[48] and Prodromos and colleagues[51] both found MRI to be more accurate than plain radiography. However, Shaffer and colleagues[48] found that only 35% of images measured within 2 mm of actual meniscus dimensions. The authors also demonstrated variability in menisci from opposite knees in the same person using MRI. Prodromos and colleagues[51] found that 94% of menisci had sagittal and coronal dimensions that were within 2 mm of the contralateral meniscus. The authors believe that their results are more accurate than those of Shaffer and colleagues, because they used a sagittal and coronal method rather than a transverse method. Donahue and colleagues[47] recently developed an algorithm for allograft sizing based on allograft parameter values and MRI scans of the uninjured knee.

Little is known about the tolerance of the tibiofemoral compartment to meniscus size mismatch. Dienst and colleagues[52] found that oversized lateral meniscal allografts led to greater forces across the articular cartilage, whereas undersized allografts resulted in normal forces across the articular cartilage but greater forces across the meniscus. The authors suggested that a mismatch in graft size of less than 10% of the size of the original meniscus may be acceptable. Haut Donahue and colleagues[53] demonstrated that both the transverse and cross-sectional width and depth are important parameters of the menisci. They found that medial meniscal parameters had a greater effect on the contact variables than the lateral meniscus and should, therefore, have more strict size tolerances. However, further studies are required to improve the reliability of graft sizing and to define the tolerance to size mismatch.

The senior author (S.A.R.) currently uses plain radiographs (taken with a size marker to aid in correcting for magnification) and MRI to determine tibial plateau dimensions. For use of a fresh-frozen graft, a matching tibial plateau (or hemi-plateau) graft with attached meniscus is obtained from the tissue bank. However, if the tissue bank supplies only the meniscus (fresh or cryopreserved allografts), it will be necessary to use some formula to derive meniscus dimensions from the bone measurements. It is recommended that the clinician become familiar with the technique used at the tissue bank supplying the grafts. Careful attention should be paid to obtaining a properly sized graft.

SURGICAL TECHNIQUE

Both open and arthroscopically assisted techniques have been described for meniscus allograft transplantation and have been reported with comparable results.[20,22,44,54] The proper selection of anchoring sites for the anterior and posterior horns, however, is likely of greater importance than the surgical technique. It is essential that the clinician is familiar with normal meniscus anatomy and the relationship of the insertion sites to other intra-articular structures, including the tibial spines and cruciate ligaments. The horn insertion sites can often be identified by a small stump of remaining meniscus (**Fig. 2**).

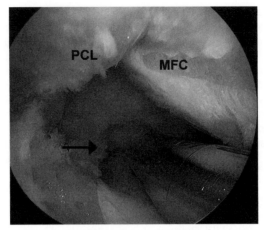

Fig. 2. It is critical to accurately identify the anatomic horn insertion sites. In this case, a small stump of remaining meniscus (*arrow*) represents the posterior horn insertion site.

There is disagreement in the literature over the best method of fixation for the meniscus allograft. Some authors have advocated suture fixation through transosseous tunnels.[28,55,56] However, cadaver models[10,57–59] suggest that implantation with attached bone results in a more secure anchorage of the horn attachment sites. These studies found superior load transmission with meniscal horn bone plug fixation compared with no bone plugs. Clinical support of this was reported by Rodeo[20] who found an 88% success rate with bone fixation compared with a 47% success rate in those without bone fixation. Sekiya and colleagues[60] also demonstrated better clinical results with bone fixation than suture fixation. The graft can be inserted with separate bone plugs attached to each horn[61] (**Fig. 3**). The diameter of the bone plugs is typically 9 mm. Using smaller bone plugs is not recommended, because they may fracture

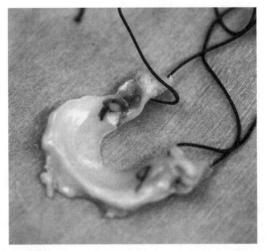

Fig. 3. Medial meniscus allograft transplant with bone plugs attached to the anterior and posterior horns. These bone plugs are transplanted into bone tunnels at the anterior and posterior horn attachment sites.

upon insertion of the graft. Alternatively, the bone slot technique[62] uses a graft with a common bone bridge that is attached to both the anterior and posterior horns. This bone bridge is then inserted into a similarly shaped slot in the recipient tibia (**Fig. 4**).

Recommended Technique for MMT

The use of bone plugs for medial transplants is currently recommended. A standard anterior cruciate ligament (ACL) or posterior cruciate ligament (PCL) guide is used to drill the tunnel for the posterior horn bone plug. The anterior horn tunnel may be drilled antegrade, with arthroscopic visualization, through a slightly enlarged anterior portal. A blind-ended tunnel is drilled in this fashion, after which a small drill hole is made from the tibial surface into the base of this tunnel to pull the sutures through. Placing the graft into the knee through an enlarged anterior portal is recommended. When passing the graft into the posterior horn tunnel, it is helpful to remove small amounts of bone from both the medial tibial spine and the inner aspect of the medial femoral condyle (analogous to performing a notchplasty). An arthroscopic probe is used to hold up the PCL to allow the meniscus to pass posteriorly into the posterior horn tunnel. A long meniscal repair needle with an attached suture is passed through the posterior portion of the graft, then through the posteromedial capsule, and retrieved via the posteromedial capsular exposure, which will be used later for meniscal suturing. This suture aids in insertion of the graft into the posterior compartment by providing a vector to pull the graft posteriorly. If graft passage is difficult in a tight medial compartment, a partial release of the medial collateral ligament (MCL) can be easily performed through the small anterior incision that is already present for the bone tunnels. This is only infrequently required. Arthroscopic sectioning of the deep MCL is not recommended, because it causes the capsule to "balloon out," which can make later meniscal suturing difficult. The sutures attached to the horns are then tied together over a bone bridge over the anterior tibia.

Some authors recommend bringing the meniscus into the knee through a posterior capsular incision to avoid the difficulty of inserting the graft into the posterior tunnel.[50]

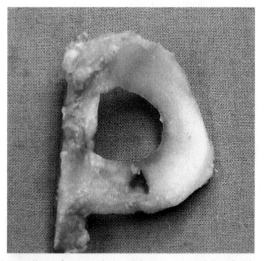

Fig. 4. Lateral meniscus allograft transplant with a common bone bridge attached to both the anterior and posterior horns.

The senior author has not found this necessary and prefers to leave the posterior capsule intact to aid in later meniscal suturing. Others have recommended avoiding bone plugs on the posterior horn of the graft to ease insertion into the posterior tunnel. The use of bone plugs on both horns is preferred to ensure secure fixation. The graft must also be securely sutured to the capsule using standard meniscal repair techniques. The senior author uses an inside-out technique with nonabsorbable, vertical mattress sutures to suture the posterior aspect and mid-body. The anterior part of the transplant can often be sutured under direct visualization via the small anterior incision (**Fig. 5**). A posterior incision is used for placement of a retractor to protect the posterior neurovascular structures during the inside-out suture placement. Use of absorbable meniscal fixation devices may be considered, but studies have demonstrated that the holding strength of these devices is inferior to that of vertical mattress sutures.[63,64]

If concomitant ACL reconstruction is performed with MMT, the starting point for the ACL tibial tunnel on the outside of the tibia is moved slightly more medially to allow central placement of the 2 smaller tunnels for the anterior and posterior horn meniscus bone plugs. Attempts should be made to avoid confluence of the ACL tibial tunnel and the anterior horn meniscus tunnel.

Recommended Technique for Lateral Meniscus Transplantation

The use of a common bone slot containing the anterior and posterior horn attachments is recommended for lateral meniscus transplants. Under direct arthroscopic visualization, the recipient slot in the tibia is created with an arthroscopic burr and small osteotomes. Special care should be taken when drilling the slot to remain central, to prevent ACL damage and avoid making the slot too far into the respective compartment (**Fig. 6**). The graft is then inserted through a small arthrotomy. Drill holes may be made from the outside, into the base of the recipient trough. Sutures placed through the bone slot are then retrieved through the drill holes and tied over the anterior tibia. Such supplemental suture fixation is not required if a trapezoidal slot with an interference fit is used. Standard arthroscopic meniscal suturing is then performed as described earlier for MMT.

For combined lateral meniscus transplantation and ACL reconstruction, the graft with a common bone slot is implanted first. The ACL tibial tunnel is then reamed. This tunnel may partially violate the meniscus bone slot, but the overall integrity of

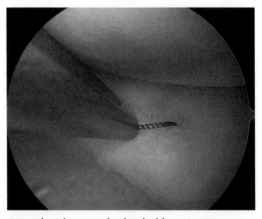

Fig. 5. The meniscus transplant is secured using inside-out sutures.

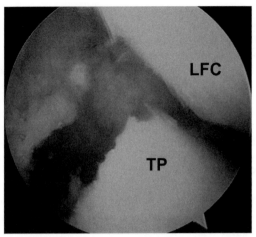

Fig. 6. The tibial slot is drilled under direct arthroscopic visualization. Care is taken to prevent injury to the ACL. Proper placement of the slot is essential to reproduce the biomechanical function of the native meniscus.

the slot usually remains intact. Alternatively, the clinician may consider staging the ACL reconstruction and lateral meniscus transplantation or use the separate bone plug technique, as described for MMT. If both medial and lateral transplants are being performed, an arthrotomy is used and the grafts are implanted with a common bone bridge containing the attachments of both menisci.

RESULTS OF MENISCUS TRANSPLANTATION

Most reports in the literature on the results of meniscal transplantation describe small case series using clinical outcome measures and/or incomplete direct evaluation of the meniscus. Therefore, results have been difficult to interpret and compare due to many confounding variables. Among them are varied methods of graft fixation and graft processing, degrees of arthrosis, indications, concomitant procedures, and definitions of failure. As a result, the study patients are a heterogeneous group. Further, there is no "gold-standard" clinical outcome measure to evaluate meniscal transplants, leading to the use of numerous different clinical grading scales (Lysholm, modified Hospital for Special Surgery [HSS] score, IKDC, "Cincinnati score," Western Ontario and McMaster Universities Osteoarthritis Index [WOMAC], Tegner, Knee Injury and Osteoarthritis Outcome Score [KOOS]) in the literature. Recently, studies have been reported with long-term follow-up and direct meniscal evaluation. Still, most provide level IV evidence and lack a control group. Although many studies include postoperative radiographs, MRI, second-look arthroscopy, and/or histologic analysis of biopsy specimens, most data are incomplete, and the study numbers are too small to draw any firm conclusions.

The clinical success of meniscus transplantation has been well documented. Numerous studies have demonstrated statistically significant improvements in pain and function using various clinical outcome measures.[15,17–22,26,28,29,42,55,60,62,65–70] This review focuses on recently published reports with long-term follow-up, direct meniscal evaluation, and large study groups, as well as those with combined procedures and isolated transplant groups.

Comparing different studies in the literature is difficult because the majority of patients have undergone concomitant procedures with meniscus transplantation. It is impossible to determine whether the clinical improvement is due to the replaced meniscus, the concomitant procedure, or both. Therefore, the most informative studies about the status and role of the meniscal allograft are those that evaluate isolated transplants and use methods such as MRI or arthroscopy to directly evaluate the meniscus.

Potter and colleagues[15] demonstrated that MRI provides accurate assessment of meniscal position, horn and capsular attachments, meniscal degeneration, and adjacent articular cartilage. The authors also found that MRI correlates well with arthroscopic evaluation of the transplant. In a sheep model of meniscal allograft transplantation, Kelly and colleagues[71] found significant correlations between T2-mapping data and all other traditional outcome measures. Kim and Bin[72] found that MRI examination correlated well with arthroscopy findings. However, other authors have failed to find a correlation between direct evaluation of the meniscus (MRI and arthroscopy) and clinical outcome.[19,22,28,38]

The outcome of meniscal transplantation may be best evaluated by analysis of isolated meniscal transplants, but very few reports exist. In many series, isolated transplants are not clearly identified or distinguished by a separate analysis. The 2 largest series of isolated lateral transplants were reported by Sekiya and colleagues[60] and van Arkel and de Boer.[17] Sekiya and colleagues[60] reported a minimum 2-year retrospective study of 25 isolated cryopreserved lateral allograft transplants. Radiographic analysis of 20 patients revealed no difference in joint-space narrowing between the involved and uninvolved knees. The radiographic joint-space measurements of the involved lateral compartment were associated with subjective assessment, symptoms, sports activity scores, Lysholm scores, and final IKDC scores. Four of the 11 patients in the bone fixation group had a normal or nearly normal overall IKDC score, compared with 0 of 6 patients with suture fixation alone.

Van Arkel and de Boer[17] reported clinical follow-up at a minimum of 2 years for 25 cryopreserved transplants and performed arthroscopic evaluation in 12 of the transplants. Partial detachment was found in 5 menisci, and 3 of these were eventually removed. There were signs of degeneration in 5 transplants. There was no change in the articular surfaces. Standing radiographs made from hip to ankle for assessment of mechanical axis demonstrated no change in 18 patients and improvement in 5 patients.

Kim and Bin[72] reported on 14 lateral allografts following resection of torn discoid lateral menisci. Osteochondral autograft transfer was performed in 3 patients for osteochondritis dissecans in the lateral femoral condyle. At a mean follow-up of 4.8 years (range, 1.75–8.75 years), the modified Lysholm score significantly improved from 71.4 to 91.4 points. Radiographs in 11 patients revealed no significant joint-space changes. MRI results in 13 patients demonstrated secure integration of the graft. Six second-look arthroscopies revealed 4 normal menisci, 1 anterior horn shrinkage, and 1 radial tear at the posterior horn (the only failure). The authors found that MRI examination correlated well with arthroscopy findings. In a study of 39 patients, Cole and colleagues[73] identified a subgroup of 21 isolated allografts. Significant improvements were identified in Lysholm, IKDC, and pain scores at minimum 2-year follow-up. Patients were completely or mostly satisfied in 81% of cases. There were no significant differences in mean preoperative or mean follow-up scores between the isolated and combined subgroups.

The review of larger series and those with direct evaluation of the meniscus provides important information on the results of meniscal transplants, which will aid in refining the indications. Milachowski and colleagues[68] were the first to report on the outcome of meniscus transplantation. The authors reported on 22 transplants (16 lyophilized, 6 fresh-frozen) with concomitant ACL reconstruction at an average follow-up of 14 months. Evaluation by arthroscopy and/or arthrography demonstrated 3 (14%) failures. The fresh-frozen transplants appeared more normal than the lyophilized menisci, which displayed shrinkage. Wirth and colleagues[42] published long-term results (14-year follow-up) and found that the group with the deep-frozen transplants was superior in clinical, radiographic, MRI, and arthroscopy results. MRI evaluation demonstrated an abnormal signal in all 6 lyophilized grafts, whereas there was normal signal in all 3 deep-frozen grafts. There was a decline in the Lysholm scores from 82 ± 15 points at 3 years to 74 ± 23 points at 14 years, and radiographs demonstrated an increase in degenerative changes of 1 grade according to Fairbank's criteria. In a comparison between the study group and 2 control groups (ACL reconstruction with either deficient menisci or intact menisci), no significant differences were found. Von Lewinski and colleagues[74] reported the 20-year results of 5 deep-frozen grafts. Lysholm scores continued to decrease over time to 74.2 ± 32 points at 20-year follow-up. Radiological results demonstrated signs of varus deformity in all patients as well as clear degenerative changes. The subjective, clinical, radiological, and MRI outcome measures showed gradual deterioration of the transplants over time. It should be noted that these transplants were done via arthrotomy, and many knees likely had pre-existing degenerative joint disease.

Noyes and colleagues[22,38] described the results of 96 consecutive fresh-frozen, irradiated transplants in 82 patients. Many of the patients underwent concomitant ACL reconstruction. All patients had direct evaluation of the transplant with either MRI or arthroscopy. Of the total 96 transplants, 56 (58%) failed, 30 (31%) were partially healed, 9 (9%) healed, and 1 (1%) was unknown. Twenty-nine of the 56 failures were removed before the minimum 2-year follow-up. There were no differences in pain or function score improvements between patients with healed or failed transplants. The high failure rate may be attributed to the relatively high-grade arthrosis present preoperatively as well as possible irradiation-induced weakening of the meniscus grafts. Failure was found to be related to joint degeneration as graded by MRI. The failure rate ranged from 6% (1 of 18 knees) in normal to mildly arthritic knees to 80% (12 of 15) in knees with advanced arthritis. The relationship between the failure rate and severity of arthrosis was significant ($P<.001$).

Verdonk and colleagues[28] recently published the results of a long-term (minimum 10 year), prospective study of 42 meniscal allograft transplants in 41 patients. All of the degenerative changes were focal, and 67% were greater than grade II. Viable allografts were transplanted via arthrotomy using a suture technique in all cases. There were 7 failures (18% failure rate), which was defined as conversion to total knee arthroplasty. The clinical outcome scores excluded the failed transplants. Modified HSS scores demonstrated significant improvements in pain and function in all subgroups. At final follow-up, 90% of all patients were satisfied with the outcome and would consider the procedure again. However, the KOOS scores (n = 25) revealed substantial disability and symptoms as well as reduced quality of life. Radiographic analysis revealed no further joint-space narrowing in 13 of 32 knees (41%) and stable Fairbank changes in 9 of 32 knees (28%). MRI analysis in nonfailure cases showed no progression of cartilage degeneration in 6 of 17 knees (35%). There was an increased signal intensity of the allograft and partial graft extrusion in the majority of patients at the final follow-up. The radiographic and MRI parameters did not correlate with the clinical outcome. Further, the status of cartilage degeneration did not correlate with clinical outcome for any group at either the time of transplantation or final follow-up.

Noyes and colleagues[19] studied 40 cryopreserved meniscal allografts in 38 patients for a mean 3.3-year follow-up. There were 16 concomitant osteoarticular transfer system (OATS) procedures and 9 concomitant ligament reconstructions. Pain with daily activities decreased from 79% to 11% of patients. Thirty-four (89%) patients rated the knee condition as improved (Cincinnati score), and 68% had no tibiofemoral pain. No differences were found between isolated transplants and combined procedure groups. Radiographs showed further deterioration and joint-space narrowing in 3 knees. There was a 44% failure rate among patients who initially had moderate arthrosis compared with 14% in those with mild arthrosis. MRI in 29 cases demonstrated a mean allograft displacement of 2.2 mm under loaded imaging conditions, and nearly all had signal intensity alterations. The authors used a rating system combining subjective, clinical, and weight-bearing MRI factors to determine meniscal allograft characteristics after implantation. A "normal" knee required all 6 criteria to be met, whereas a "failed" knee required only 1 failed criterion. Meniscal allograft characteristics were normal in 17 knees (43%), altered in 12 (30%), and failed in 11 (28%). However, there was no correlation between allograft characteristics and score for patient perception of the knee condition. Concomitant OATS and stabilization procedures had similar improvements and did not increase the rate of complications.

Rodeo[20] reported on 33 fresh-frozen, nonirradiated meniscus transplants at a minimum 2-year follow-up. The patients were evaluated with MRI and/or arthroscopic inspection. Preoperatively, 18 patients had grade IV and 6 patients had grade III articular degeneration. Based on the objective evaluation of the 33 total meniscal transplants, there were 8 good, 14 moderate, 4 poor, and 7 failed meniscus transplants. There was no significant change in joint degeneration at this follow-up interval. One of 6 patients with Outerbridge grade III failed, whereas 6 of 18 patients with Outerbridge grade IV changes failed. MRI and arthroscopic inspections of the meniscus transplants demonstrated consistent healing of the meniscus transplant to the capsule and at the bone-plug attachment sites. MRI showed that there was frequently some degree of extrusion of the transplant from the tibiofemoral compartment. The degree of extrusion was greatest in knees with more advanced articular degeneration (Fig. 7). MRI also demonstrated variable amounts of increased intrameniscal signal within the substance of the meniscus, which is indicative of ongoing remodeling of the transplant and/or degeneration. Increased signal was most frequently observed in the posterior horn of the meniscus, in areas where the overlying articular cartilage was thinned or absent. There were significant improvements in Lysholm, IKDC, and visual analog scale (VAS) scores. The results were significantly better for menisci that were transplanted with attached bone plugs than for those implanted without bone plugs. Fourteen out of 16 (88%) of the menisci implanted with bone plugs were rated as good or moderate, while 8 out of 17 (47%) of the menisci implanted without bone plugs were rated as good or moderate ($P = .03$). Three out of the 7 failed allografts had been implanted with attached bone plugs.

In 2006, Cole and colleagues[73] reported a prospective study of 44 meniscus transplants in 39 patients with a minimum 2-year follow-up (mean, 2.8 years). Lysholm scores improved from 52.4 to 71.6, and IKDC scores improved from 46.2 to 64.1. Patients were classified as normal or nearly normal using the IKDC score in 90% of cases at final follow-up. No significant differences were detected between the medial and lateral subgroups, although the lateral transplants demonstrated a trend toward greater improvement on most knee scoring scales. At final follow-up, 7 patients had failed (16% failure rate). The study did not include any direct evaluation of the transplant.

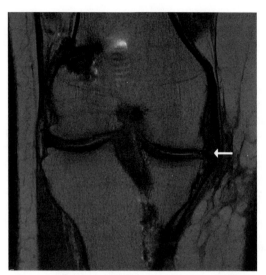

Fig. 7. Extrusion is usually associated with degeneration of the meniscus adjacent to the posterior horn attachment. In this case, a coronal MRI image demonstrates extrusion of the body segment of the medial meniscal transplant.

Verdonk and colleagues[29] reported a survivorship analysis and clinical outcomes of 100 viable meniscal allograft transplants after a mean of 7.2 years (range, 0.5–14.5 years). All grafts were transplanted using suture fixation of the horn attachment sites. Overall, pain scores improved from 13.7 to 39.4 (out of 50), and function scores improved from 60.1 to 88.6 (modified HSS scores). There were 21 failures, which were defined as moderate occasional or persistent pain or as poor function. The mean cumulative survival time was 11.6 years and was identical for the medial and lateral groups. The cumulative survival rates for the medial and lateral allografts at 10 years were 74.2% and 69.8% respectively. Stone and colleagues[57] reported a prospective study using 47 allografts with an average 5.8-year (range, 2–7.25 years) follow-up. When compared with most other studies, the patients were older (mean age, 48 years; range, 14–69 years) and had more advanced arthrosis (all patients, grade III or IV; 81%, grade IV). All patients had concomitant procedures. Twenty-nine grafts (62%) were cryopreserved, and 18 (38%) were fresh-frozen. There were significant improvements in subjective outcome measures (IKDC, WOMAC, and Tegner), but no difference was detected between groups with different concomitant procedures. There were 5 failures (10.6%) with a mean failure time of 4.4 years. All failures were observed in Outerbridge grade IV patients, and 4 failures were with cryopreserved grafts. The best predictor of failure was the number of previous surgeries. Given that the results among this older, more arthritic patient group compared favorably with outcomes in younger patients without degenerative disease, the authors suggested that the existing contraindications based on age and arthrosis severity may be overstated. However, there was no direct inspection or imaging of the transplants.

In 2007, Hommen and colleagues[75] published the results of 20 cryopreserved meniscus allograft transplants at a mean follow-up of 11.8 years (range, 9.6–13.9 years). Twenty-four concomitant procedures were performed in 15 patients. There were significant improvements in mean Lysholm (53–75) and pain (4.8–2.4) scores, which improved in 90% of patients. Ten of the 15 patients with follow-up radiographs had progressive joint-space narrowing of the involved compartment from 5.15 mm to 4 mm (P = .0002). Twelve of the 15 patients showed progression of the Fairbank grade of degenerative joint disease (0.5–1.3, P = .0001). The radiographic changes correlated with lower postoperative Lysholm scores. Five of 7 patients who underwent MRI had a grade III tear of the posterior horn of the allograft with associated clinical signs. The authors reported failures in 11 of the 20 patients (55%), with failure defined as known surgical failures, unimproved patient knee survey scores, and MRI failures.

Several studies have focused on the results of meniscal allograft transplants combined with other procedures such as ligament reconstruction, chondral resurfacing, and osteotomy. Many authors have attempted to compare the results of isolated transplants, transplants combined with other procedures, and various combinations of different procedures. Although all of these groups have shown improvement, there have not been significant differences in important outcome measures.[19,23,25,36,55,75]

Meniscal Transplant Combined with ACL Reconstruction

Rueff and colleagues[36] reported a case-controlled series of ACL reconstructions with either meniscus transplants (group 1) or partial meniscectomy or meniscal repair (group 2). Each group had 8 patients who were matched for age, sex, and activity level. Both groups displayed similar improvements in modified Lysholm and IKDC scores (P<.05), but the transplant group displayed greater pain improvement.

Graf and colleagues[67] reported the long-term (mean, 9.7 years) results of 8 medial meniscal allograft transplantations combined with ACL reconstruction. All grafts were cryopreserved (7 irradiated at 3.0 Mrad; 1 not irradiated). Consistent with previous short-term follow-up reports, there was improvement in pain, swelling, stability, and knee function. All 8 patients would recommend the procedure to a friend and would undergo the procedure again. Six patients had a second-look arthroscopy (3 at >6-year follow-up; 3 at <1.5-year follow-up). There was no graft shrinkage and a 100% survival rate, with each graft completely healed to the capsule. There was a small tear in 1 graft from a new twisting injury, and a loose body was found in 1 knee.

Meniscal Transplant Combined with Chondral Resurfacing

Rue and colleagues[23] reported a prospective study of 29 meniscal transplants combined with chondral resurfacing procedures with a mean follow-up of 3.1 years (range, 1.9–5.6 years). There were 15 autologous chondrocyte implants (ACIs) (mean lesion size, 3.93 cm^2) and 14 OAs (size, 5.48 cm^2). All groups had statistically significant improvements in all subjective outcome scores except for the SF-12 mental score. Although the absolute outcome scores were significantly better for the ACI group versus the OA group, the percentage improvement from the pre-operative scores did not differ significantly. There was no difference in outcomes between the medial and lateral groups. There were 2 failures, which was defined as revision or arthroscopic confirmation of failure of either procedure. In the most recent follow-up, 48% were classified as normal or nearly normal using the IKDC score. Seventy-six percent of all patients were completely (31%) or mostly (45%) satisfied with their results, and 90% would choose to have the surgery again. The authors concluded that the results of the combined procedures were comparable to published reports of these procedures performed in isolation. The combined procedure groups did not have an increase in complication rate.

Farr and colleagues[25] reported the minimum 2-year follow-up results of 33 cases of combined meniscal transplant and ACI. Sixteen patients had additional concomitant procedures performed. Four grafts failed before the 2-year follow-up and were excluded from analysis. The mean Browne modified Cincinnati score improved from 3.96 to 6.29, and the Lysholm score improved from 57.7 to 77.7.

Bhosale and colleagues[24] studied a consecutive series of 8 meniscal transplants combined with ACIs (for large kissing chondral defects). The meniscus grafts were cryopreserved and inserted with bone plugs. Six of the 8 patients reported improved pain relief and function at 1 year. The midterm results (mean, 3.2 years; range, 2–6 years) demonstrated functional improvement in 5 of the 8 patients. There were 3 failures, although 1 was in a patient aged 58 years with multiple previous surgeries. MRI results in 5 patients showed good integration of menisci with the capsule, without any rejection, and mild extrusion in 1 case (clinically asymptomatic). The replaced chondral surfaces were irregular, possibly reflecting fibrillation of the surface with variable graft thicknesses. Arthroscopy in 8 cases showed a stable meniscus with healed peripheral margins in all patients except 1. Two cases exhibited mild synovitis. Histologic analysis of biopsy specimens in all 8 meniscal implants confirmed fibrocartilage that was well populated with viable cells, some of which appeared to be proliferating. The ACI grafts were well integrated with underlying bone.

Axial Alignment

The importance of neutral axial alignment on the outcome of meniscus transplantation has been demonstrated by several studies. Verdonk and colleagues[28] reported the long-term results (minimum, 10 years) on 27 MMTs. Eleven of these transplants also underwent an HTO (MMT + HTO) to correct varus malalignment of the lower limb. The MMT + HTO group had significantly better improvements in pain (Modified HSS score, KOOS) and function (KOOS) than the MMT group. MRI evaluation demonstrated fewer grafts with grade III signal in the MMT + HTO group. Verdonk and colleagues[29] also performed a survivorship analysis of viable meniscal allograft transplants after a mean of 7.2 years. The 10-year survival rates were 83.3% for the MMT + HTO group compared with 74.2% for the MMT group.

Van Arkel and de Boer[17] reported on 23 cryopreserved transplants at a minimum 2-year follow-up. All 3 failures (transplant removed) were found to be related to malalignment. The scores on standardized knee scales (Lysholm and Knee Assessment Scoring System) were higher for patients with neutral alignment. Cameron and Saha[26] reported on 34 knees that received a meniscal allograft in combination with osteotomy (valgus high tibial, varus high tibial, or varus distal femoral). Good or excellent results were found in 29 (85%) of these patients. These authors acknowledged the difficulty in determining which part of the procedure was most important in providing clinical improvement.

Medial versus Lateral Transplants

Many series have attempted to compare the success of MMT with that of lateral transplants. Most have failed to find any significant differences,[23,25,28,29,73,75] although several studies have found that lateral transplants survive longer and have better clinical results.[19,76] Van Arkel and colleagues[76] reported a survival analysis of 63 meniscal allograft transplants in 57 patients for an average of 5 years (range, 0.3–10.5 years). The cumulative survival rates for lateral, medial, and combined meniscal transplants were 76%, 50%, and 67%, respectively. The lateral allografts lasted longer and had fewer failures than the medial allografts.

Graft Processing

Different grafts are used for meniscus transplant, most commonly cryopreserved[19,24,36,60,67] and fresh frozen.[20,74] Lyophilized grafts have been found to be inferior to deep-frozen grafts in arthroscopic appearance and clinical results and are no longer recommended.[42,68] Verdonk and colleagues[28] transplanted 42 fresh menisci in 41 patients with a minimum 10-year follow-up. MRI evaluation showed that the position of the graft was unchanged in 6 of 17 knees, progressive extrusion occurred in 10 of 17 knees, and only a small remnant of the graft was present in 1 knee. Zukor and colleagues[77] transplanted 28 fresh menisci as part of a tibial plateau OA. Direct evaluation with arthroscopy or arthrotomy was performed for 14 transplants. The grafts were found to be structurally intact and well attached. There were degenerative changes and small tears seen in some, but none required removal. It is difficult to draw definitive conclusions regarding the role of graft processing on the clinical outcome based on the current literature. Small patient numbers and the numerous confounding variables are a likely explanation for the lack of significant differences between different graft types.

MECHANISMS OF FAILURE OF MENISCUS TRANSPLANTS

Several factors may contribute to the failure of meniscus transplants, which include biomechanics, biological factors, surgical technique, and proper graft sizing. The principal factor involved in failure appears to be advanced articular cartilage degeneration, which likely results in excessive stresses on the transplanted meniscus. The presence of osseous remodeling of the tibiofemoral compartment, with flattening of the femoral condyle, is associated with degeneration of the meniscus. Noyes and Barber-Westin[22] found that failure of meniscus transplants correlated with the flattening of the femoral condyles on MRI. Degeneration and tears most commonly occur adjacent to the posterior horn attachment, where the contact stresses on the meniscus are highest (**Fig. 8**). Improper placement of anterior and posterior horn fixation sites will likely adversely affect the biomechanical function of the meniscus. The tolerance for graft size mismatch is not known. Undersized grafts result in increased forces across the meniscus, and oversized grafts lead to greater articular cartilage stresses.[52]

Biologic factors also likely play a role in failure of meniscal transplants. Rodeo and colleagues[78] used immunohistochemistry and routine histology to examine biopsies of meniscus and synovium from patients with both intact and failed transplants. Although frank immune rejection did not appear to occur, there was microscopic evidence of an immune response against the transplant. Such a subclinical immune response may contribute to graft shrinkage and persistent effusions. There was incomplete cellular repopulation, with more cells at the periphery (**Fig. 9**). The central area often remained hypocellular or acellular. The repopulating cells had several phenotypes: mononuclear/synovial cells, fibroblasts, and fibrochondrocytes. There was active matrix remodeling by the repopulating cells. This remodeling process may weaken the tissue and predispose to tears and graft failure. Further information about the cellular repopulation process will aid in the understanding of graft healing and graft incorporation.

REHABILITATION

The principles used for rehabilitation after meniscus repair can provide some guidance for determining the ideal postoperative management of meniscal allograft transplantation. The loads placed on the healing meniscal allograft during rehabilitation activities are unknown. However, since meniscal transplants are thought to be under higher

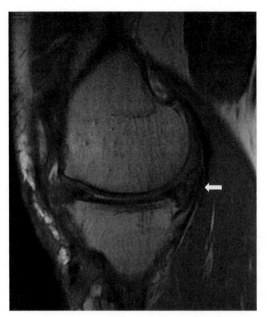

Fig. 8. Contact stresses on the menisci are highest in the posterior horn, which may result in degeneration or tears. This MRI demonstrates the degeneration in the posterior horn of a transplanted meniscus.

stresses in a joint with early degenerative changes, a more conservative protocol is typically recommended.

The senior author's current postoperative protocol involves use of a standard double-upright, hinged knee brace for the first 6 weeks. Only toe-touch weight bearing with the knee in full extension is allowed for the first 4 weeks, with gradual progression to full weight bearing by 6 weeks postoperatively. Early range-of-motion exercise is begun immediately, including full extension. Flexion is limited to 90° during the first 4 weeks because progressive knee flexion subjects the meniscus to greater stress.[5]

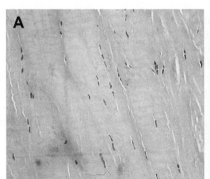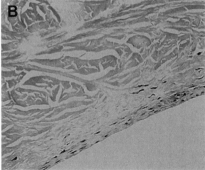

Fig. 9. *A*: Histologic section of normal meniscus, with fibrochondrocytes evenly distributed throughout the tissue. *B*: Biopsy of a human meniscus allograft 6 mo after transplantation demonstrates incomplete cellular repopulation. There are cells in the superficial aspect of the meniscus, whereas the deeper layer remains acellular.

This is supported by the observation by Morgan and colleagues[32] that extension appears to reduce the meniscus to the capsule whereas flexion causes posterior horn tears to displace from the capsule. In addition, Thompson and colleagues[79] demonstrated that the menisci translate posteriorly with flexion; however, meniscal movement was minimal below 60° of flexion. No significant flexion limitations have occurred using this protocol.

Range of motion is progressed after 4 to 6 weeks. Closed kinetic chain strengthening exercises within the flexion limits are begun in the third week and progressed. Fritz and colleagues[80] suggest avoidance of early open-chain knee flexion exercises due to the attachment of the semimembranosus on the medial meniscus and the popliteus on the lateral meniscus. Gentle sport-specific activities are initiated after 4 months for further development of strength and proprioception. Running is not recommended before 4 months. Squatting and hyperflexion are discouraged for 6 months following meniscal transplantation. Return to high-load activities involving cutting, jumping, and pivoting are determined on an individual basis. If there was concomitant ACL reconstruction, the usual ACL rehabilitation protocol is modified as described here. Early full extension is emphasized. Concomitant cartilage resurfacing procedures may also require modifications in the postoperative program. The senior author also considers use of an unloader brace to protect the allograft for the first 4 to 6 weeks after the patient resumes weight bearing (weeks 7–12).

FUTURE MENISCAL REPLACEMENT IMPLANTS

Future meniscal replacement alternatives will benefit from the experience with meniscal allograft transplantation. These future options include tissue-engineered menisci,[81] bioactive scaffolds,[82–84] and synthetic devices.[85–87] The Collagen Meniscus Implant (CMI [now called Menaflex]; ReGen Biologics, Hackensack, New Jersey) is a scaffold designed to support new tissue formation. The implant requires a meniscal rim for attachment and, therefore, can only fill partial meniscal defects. In a prospective randomized study, Rodkey and colleagues[83] found that patients with chronic meniscal injury who received the CMI regained significantly more of their lost activity compared with patients with only repeat partial meniscectomy. However, the effect of CMI on meniscal function remains unknown and requires long-term assessment of degenerative changes.[88] Another scaffold material that is currently under investigation in humans is bioresorbable porous polyurethane.[84]

Hydrogel meniscal implants are synthetic devices that are durable in small animal models.[86,87] Kelly and coworkers[85] demonstrated that hydrogel meniscal replacement (Salumedica, Inc, Atlanta, Georgia) in an ovine model leads to significantly decreased cartilage degeneration compared with meniscectomy. However, the animals that received a hydrogel implant had significantly increased cartilage degeneration in the peripheral tibial plateau when compared with meniscal allograft transplantation. While these studies suggest a protective role for hydrogel implants in the short to intermediate term, the long-term results are still unknown. Further options for meniscus replacement or regeneration may arise from advancements in fields such as biomaterials, gene therapy, and stem cell biology.

SUMMARY

Meniscal allograft transplantation has emerged as a treatment option for selected meniscus-deficient patients to restore normal meniscal function and forestall progressive joint degeneration. Concomitant procedures, such as chondral resurfacing, osteotomy, and ligament reconstruction, may render a knee suitable for meniscal transplantation and increase graft survival. However, further study with direct evaluation of the transplanted meniscus is required to better define the indications and outcomes of such combined procedures. Mid- and long-term reports have demonstrated predictable improvements in pain, swelling, and knee function with meniscal allograft transplantation. Despite these clinical improvements, there is still minimal evidence that meniscal allografts improve or restore meniscal function. This information will only be known with long-term assessment of degenerative changes with direct evaluation of the meniscus. Further understanding of the biology of transplants will also refine the use of this technique. Future meniscal replacement options may include tissue-engineered menisci, bioactive scaffolds, and synthetic implants.

REFERENCES

1. Levy IM, Torzilli PA, Warren RF. The effect of medial meniscectomy on anterior-posterior motion of the knee. J Bone Joint Surg Am 1982;64:883–8.
2. Allen CR, Wong EK, Livesay GA, et al. Importance of the medial meniscus in the anterior cruciate ligament-deficient knee. J Orthop Res 2000;18:109–15.
3. Levy IM, Torzilli PA, Gould JD, et al. The effect of lateral meniscectomy on motion of the knee. J Bone Joint Surg Am 1989;71:401–6.
4. Shelbourne KD, Gray T. Results of anterior cruciate ligament reconstruction based on meniscus and articular cartilage status at the time of surgery. Five- to fifteen-year evaluations. Am J Sports Med 2000;28:446–52.
5. Walker PS, Erkman MJ. The role of the menisci in force transmission across the knee. Clin Orthop Relat Res 1975;184–92.
6. Fairbank TJ. Knee joint changes after Meniscectomy. J Bone Joint Surg Br 1948; 30:664–70.
7. Cox JS, Nye CE, Schaefer WW, et al. The degenerative effects of partial and total resection of the medial meniscus in dogs' knees. Clin Orthop Relat Res 1975;178–83.
8. Kurosawa H, Fukubayashi T, Nakajima H. Load-bearing mode of the knee joint: physical behavior of the knee joint with or without menisci. Clin Orthop Relat Res 1980;283–90.
9. Baratz ME, Fu FH, Mengato R. Meniscal tears: the effect of meniscectomy and of repair on intraarticular contact areas and stress in the human knee. A preliminary report. Am J Sports Med 1986;14:270–5.
10. McDermott ID, Lie DT, Edwards A, et al. The effects of lateral meniscal allograft transplantation techniques on tibio-femoral contact pressures. Knee Surg Sports Traumatol Arthrosc 2008;16:553–60.
11. Yocum LA, Kerlan RK, Jobe FW, et al. Isolated lateral meniscectomy. A study of twenty-six patients with isolated tears. J Bone Joint Surg Am 1979;61:338–42.
12. Johnson RJ, Kettelkamp DB, Clark W, et al. Factors effecting late results after meniscectomy. J Bone Joint Surg Am 1974;56:719–29.
13. Tapper EM, Hoover NW. Late results after meniscectomy. J Bone Joint Surg Am 1969;51:517–26.
14. Appel H. Late results after meniscectomy in the knee joint. A clinical and roentgenologic follow-up investigation. Acta Orthop Scand Suppl 1970;133:1–111.
15. Potter HG, Linklater JM, Allen AA, et al. Magnetic resonance imaging of articular cartilage in the knee. An evaluation with use of fast-spin-echo imaging. J Bone Joint Surg Am 1998;80:1276–84.
16. Dye SF, Chew MH. The use of scintigraphy to detect increased osseous metabolic activity about the knee. Instr Course Lect 1994;43:453–69.

17. van Arkel ER, de Boer HH. Human meniscal transplantation. Preliminary results at 2 to 5-year follow-up. J Bone Joint Surg Br 1995;77:589–95.

18. Garrett J. Meniscal transplantation. In: Aichroth P, Cannon W, editors. Knee Surgery: Current Practice. London: Martin Dunitz, Ltd; 1992. p. 95–103.

19. Noyes FR, Barber-Westin SD, Rankin M. Meniscal transplantation in symptomatic patients less than fifty years old. J Bone Joint Surg Am 2004;86:1392–404.

20. Rodeo SA. Meniscal allografts—where do we stand? Am J Sports Med 2001;29: 246–61.

21. Carter T. Meniscal allograft transplantation. Sports Med Arthrosc 1999;51–62.

22. Noyes FR, Barber-Westin SD. Irradiated meniscus allografts in the human knee: a two to five year follow-up study. Orthop Trans 1995;19:417.

23. Rue JP, Yanke AB, Busam ML, et al. Prospective evaluation of concurrent meniscus transplantation and articular cartilage repair: minimum 2-year follow-up. Am J Sports Med 2008;36:1770–8.

24. Bhosale AM, Myint P, Roberts S, et al. Combined autologous chondrocyte implantation and allogenic meniscus transplantation: a biological knee replacement. Knee 2007;14:361–8.

25. Farr J, Rawal A, Marberry KM. Concomitant meniscal allograft transplantation and autologous chondrocyte implantation: minimum 2-year follow-up. Am J Sports Med 2007;35:1459–66.

26. Cameron JC, Saha S. Meniscal allograft transplantation for unicompartmental arthritis of the knee. Clin Orthop Relat Res 1997;164–71.

27. Holden DL, James SL, Larson RL, et al. Proximal tibial osteotomy in patients who are fifty years old or less. A long-term follow-up study. J Bone Joint Surg Am 1988;70:977–82.

28. Verdonk PC, Verstraete KL, Almqvist KF, et al. Meniscal allograft transplantation: long-term clinical results with radiological and magnetic resonance imaging correlations. Knee Surg Sports Traumatol Arthrosc 2006;14:694–706.

29. Verdonk PC, Demurie A, Almqvist KF, et al. Transplantation of viable meniscal allograft. Survivorship analysis and clinical outcome of one hundred cases. J Bone Joint Surg Am 2005;87:715–24.

30. Papageorgiou CD, Gil JE, Kanamori A, et al. The biomechanical interdependence between the anterior cruciate ligament replacement graft and the medial meniscus. Am J Sports Med 2001;29:226–31.

31. Markolf KL, Kochan A, Amstutz HC. Measurement of knee stiffness and laxity in patients with documented absence of the anterior cruciate ligament. J Bone Joint Surg Am 1984;66:242–52.

32. Morgan CD, Wojtys EM, Casscells CD, et al. Arthroscopic meniscal repair evaluated by second-look arthroscopy. Am J Sports Med 1991;19:632–7 [discussion 637–8].

33. Cannon D. Meniscal healing. In: Cannon D, editor. Arthroscopic Meniscal Repair. Rosemont (IL): American Academy of Orthopaedic Surgeons; 1999. p. 7–12.

34. Shelbourne KD, Stube KC. Anterior cruciate ligament (ACL)-deficient knee with degenerative arthrosis: treatment with an isolated autogenous patellar tendon ACL reconstruction. Knee Surg Sports Traumatol Arthrosc 1997;5:150–6.

35. Noyes FR, Barber-Westin SD, Hewett TE. High tibial osteotomy and ligament reconstruction for varus angulated anterior cruciate ligament-deficient knees. Am J Sports Med 2000;28:282–96.

36. Rueff D, Nyland J, Kocabey Y, et al. Self-reported patient outcomes at a minimum of 5 years after allograft anterior cruciate ligament reconstruction with or without medial meniscus transplantation: an age-, sex-, and activity level-matched comparison in patients aged approximately 50 years. Arthroscopy 2006;22:1053–62.

37. Li G, DeFrate LE, Park SE, et al. In vivo articular cartilage contact kinematics of the knee: an investigation using dual-orthogonal fluoroscopy and magnetic resonance image-based computer models. Am J Sports Med 2005;33:102–7.
38. Noyes FR, Barber-Westin SD, Butler DL, et al. The role of allografts in repair and reconstruction of knee joint ligaments and menisci. Instr Course Lect 1998;47:379–96.
39. Rosenberg TD, Paulos LE, Parker RD, et al. The forty-five-degree posteroanterior flexion weight-bearing radiograph of the knee. J Bone Joint Surg Am 1988;70: 1479–83.
40. Jackson DW, Whelan J, Simon TM. Cell survival after transplantation of fresh meniscal allografts. DNA probe analysis in a goat model. Am J Sports Med 1993;21:540–50.
41. Fabbriciani C, Lucania L, Milano G, et al. Meniscal allografts: cryopreservation vs deep-frozen technique. An experimental study in goats. Knee Surg Sports Traumatol Arthrosc 1997;5:124–34.
42. Wirth CJ, Peters G, Milachowski KA, et al. Long-term results of meniscal allograft transplantation. Am J Sports Med 2002;30:174–81.
43. Jackson DW, Windler GE, Simon TM. Intraarticular reaction associated with the use of freeze-dried, ethylene oxide-sterilized bone-patella tendon-bone allografts in the reconstruction of the anterior cruciate ligament. Am J Sports Med 1990;18: 1–10 [discussion 10–1].
44. Yoldas EA, Irrgang J, Fu FH, et al. Arthroscopically-assisted meniscal transplantation using non-irradiated fresh-frozen menisci. Presented at Annual Meeting of the American Academy of Orthopaedic Surgeons. New Orleans, March 1998.
45. Urban WP Jr, Nyland J, Caborn DN, et al. The radiographic position of medial and lateral meniscal horns as a basis for meniscal reconstruction. Arthroscopy 1999; 15:147–54.
46. Pollard ME, Kang Q, Berg EE. Radiographic sizing for meniscal transplantation. Arthroscopy 1995;11:684–7.
47. Donahue TL, Hull ML, Howell SM. New algorithm for selecting meniscal allografts that best match the size and shape of the damaged meniscus. J Orthop Res 2006;24:1535–43.
48. Shaffer B, Kennedy S, Klimkiewicz J, et al. Preoperative sizing of meniscal allografts in meniscus transplantation. Am J Sports Med 2000;28:524–33.
49. Kuhn JE, Wojtys EM. Allograft meniscus transplantation. Clin Sports Med 1996; 15:536–7.
50. Johnson D, Swenson T, Harner C. Meniscal reconstruction using allograft tissue: an arthroscopic technique. Oper Tech Sports Med 1994;2:223–31.
51. Prodromos CC, Joyce BT, Keller BL, et al. Magnetic resonance imaging measurement of the contralateral normal meniscus is a more accurate method of determining meniscal allograft size than radiographic measurement of the recipient tibial plateau. Arthroscopy 2007;23:1174–9, e1171.
52. Dienst M, Greis PE, Ellis BJ, et al. Effect of lateral meniscal allograft sizing on contact mechanics of the lateral tibial plateau: an experimental study in human cadaveric knee joints. Am J Sports Med 2007;35:34–42.
53. Haut Donahue TL, Hull ML, Rashid MM, et al. The sensitivity of tibiofemoral contact pressure to the size and shape of the lateral and medial menisci. J Orthop Res 2004;22:807–14.
54. Peters G, Wirth CJ, Milachowski KA, et al. Long-term results of meniscal allograft transplantation. Arthroscopy 2000;11:684–7.
55. Stone KR, Walgenbach AW, Turek TJ, et al. Meniscus allograft survival in patients with moderate to severe unicompartmental arthritis: a 2- to 7-year follow-up. Arthroscopy 2006;22:469–78.

56. Boss A, Klimkiewicz J, Fu FH. Technical innovation: creation of a peripheral vascularized trough to enhance healing in cryopreserved meniscal allograft reconstruction. Knee Surg Sports Traumatol Arthrosc 2000;8:159–62.
57. Alhalki MM, Howell SM, Hull ML. How three methods for fixing a medial meniscal autograft affect tibial contact mechanics. Am J Sports Med 1999;27:320–8.
58. Chen MI, Branch TP, Hutton WC. Is it important to secure the horns during lateral meniscal transplantation? A cadaveric study. Arthroscopy 1996;12:174–81.
59. Paletta GA Jr, Manning T, Snell E, et al. The effect of allograft meniscal replacement on intraarticular contact area and pressures in the human knee. A biomechanical study. Am J Sports Med 1997;25:692–8.
60. Sekiya JK, West RV, Groff YJ, et al. Clinical outcomes following isolated lateral meniscal allograft transplantation. Arthroscopy 2006;22:771–80.
61. Shelton WR, Dukes AD. Meniscus replacement with bone anchors: a surgical technique. Arthroscopy 1994;10:324–7.
62. Goble E, Kane S, Wilcox T, et al. Meniscal allografts. In: McGinty J, Caspari R, Jackson R, et al, editors. Operative Arthroscopy. Philadelphia: Lippincott-Raven; 1996. p. 317–31.
63. Dervin GF, Downing KJ, Keene GC, et al. Failure strengths of suture versus biodegradable arrow for meniscal repair: an in vitro study. Arthroscopy 1997;13: 296–300.
64. Albrecht-Olsen P, Lind T, Kristensen G, et al. Failure strength of a new meniscus arrow repair technique: biomechanical comparison with horizontal suture. Arthroscopy 1997;13:183–7.
65. Cole BJ, Carter TR, Rodeo SA. Allograft meniscal transplantation: background, techniques, and results. Instr Course Lect 2003;52:383–96.
66. Rath E, Richmond JC, Yassir W, et al. Meniscal allograft transplantation. Two- to eight-year results. Am J Sports Med 2001;29:410–4.
67. Graf KW Jr, Sekiya JK, Wojtys EM. Long-term results after combined medial meniscal allograft transplantation and anterior cruciate ligament reconstruction: minimum 8.5-year follow-up study. Arthroscopy 2004;20:129–40.
68. Milachowski KA, Weismeier K, Wirth CJ. Homologous meniscus transplantation. Experimental and clinical results. Int Orthop 1989;13:1–11.
69. Stollsteimer GT, Shelton WR, Dukes A, et al. Meniscal allograft transplantation: a 1- to 5-year follow-up of 22 patients. Arthroscopy 2000;16:343–7.
70. Yoldas EA, Sekiya JK, Irrgang JJ, et al. Arthroscopically assisted meniscal allograft transplantation with and without combined anterior cruciate ligament reconstruction. Knee Surg Sports Traumatol Arthrosc 2003;11:173–82.
71. Kelly BT, Potter HG, Deng XH, et al. Meniscal allograft transplantation in the sheep knee: evaluation of chondroprotective effects. Am J Sports Med 2006; 34:1464–77.
72. Kim JM, Bin SI. Meniscal allograft transplantation after total meniscectomy of torn discoid lateral meniscus. Arthroscopy 2006;22:1344–50, e1341.
73. Cole BJ, Dennis MG, Lee SJ, et al. Prospective evaluation of allograft meniscus transplantation: a minimum 2-year follow-up. Am J Sports Med 2006;34:919–27.
74. von Lewinski G, Milachowski KA, Weismeier K, et al. Twenty-year results of combined meniscal allograft transplantation, anterior cruciate ligament reconstruction and advancement of the medial collateral ligament. Knee Surg Sports Traumatol Arthrosc 2007;15:1072–82.
75. Hommen JP, Applegate GR, Del Pizzo W. Meniscus allograft transplantation: ten-year results of cryopreserved allografts. Arthroscopy 2007;23:388–93.

76. van Arkel ER, de Boer HH. Survival analysis of human meniscal transplantations. J Bone Joint Surg Br 2002;84:227–31.
77. Zukor D, Brooks P, Gross A. Meniscal allograft-experimental and clinical study. Orthod Rev 1988;17:522.
78. Rodeo SA, Seneviratne A, Suzuki K, et al. Histological analysis of human meniscal allografts. A preliminary report. J Bone Joint Surg Am 2000;82:1071–82.
79. Thompson WO, Thaete FL, Fu FH, et al. Tibial meniscal dynamics using three-dimensional reconstruction of magnetic resonance images. Am J Sports Med 1991;19:210–5 [discussion 215–6].
80. Fritz JM, Irrgang JJ, Harner CD. Rehabilitation following allograft meniscal transplantation: a review of the literature and case study. J Orthop Sports Phys Ther 1996;24:98–106.
81. Hidaka C, Ibarra C, Hannafin JA, et al. Formation of vascularized meniscal tissue by combining gene therapy with tissue engineering. Tissue Eng 2002;8:93–105.
82. Rodkey WG, Steadman JR, Li ST. A clinical study of collagen meniscus implants to restore the injured meniscus. Clin Orthop 1999;367S:S281–92.
83. Rodkey WG, DeHaven KE, Montgomery WH 3rd, et al. Comparison of the collagen meniscus implant with partial meniscectomy. A prospective randomized trial. J Bone Joint Surg Am 2008;90:1413–26.
84. Ramrattan NN, Heijkants RG, van Tienen TG, et al. Assessment of tissue ingrowth rates in polyurethane scaffolds for tissue engineering. Tissue Eng 2005;11: 1212–23.
85. Kelly BT, Robertson W, Potter HG, et al. Hydrogel meniscal replacement in the sheep knee: preliminary evaluation of chondroprotective effects. Am J Sports Med 2007;35:43–52.
86. Kobayashi M, Toguchida J, Oka M. Preliminary study of polyvinyl alcohol-hydrogel (PVA-H) artificial meniscus. Biomaterials 2003;24:639–47.
87. Kobayashi M, Toguchida J, Oka M. Development of an artificial meniscus using polyvinyl alcohol-hydrogel for early return to, and continuance of, athletic life in sportspersons with severe meniscus injury. II: animal experiments. Knee 2003; 10:53.
88. Rodeo SA. Commentary on: Comparison of the collagen meniscus implant with partial meniscectomy. A prospective randomized trial. J Bone Joint Surg Am 2008;90:1413–26.

Osteochondral Allografts: State of the Art

Christian Lattermann, MD*, Spencer E. Romine, MD

KEYWORDS

- Osteochondral allograft • Osteochondral defect
- Articular cartilage • Cartilage transplantation

The use of osteochondral allografts continues to gain popularity among orthopedists; however, the concept of replacing bone defects with allograft tissue is not a novel technique. Bolano and Kopta[1] noted that MacEwen was the first to use bone allograft over 120 years ago, followed by Lexer[2] in 1908. A subsequent decline in the early twentieth century was followed by a revival in the 1970s, especially in North America.[3] Today, the use of osteochondral allografts continues to rise throughout the orthopedic world. In 2004, approximately 800,000 bone allografts were used in the United States alone.[4] According to Delloye and colleagues,[5] bone allograft is the most commonly used bone substitute in Europe. With regard to the use of osteochondral allografts for cartilage repair, it has become clear that despite the introduction of several operative procedures that attempt to repair and restore articular cartilage,[6–9] osteochondral allografting is currently the only option that can potentially restore mature hyaline cartilage in a biologically and structurally appropriate manner. Success can be attributed to advancing technology, reproducible techniques, and an enormous increase in clinical and scientific research.[9]

BASIC SCIENCE

Articular cartilage provides a less than favorable environment for healing. Lack of blood vessels, lymphatics, nerves, and cells capable of a reparative process limits nature's ability to restore lesions of the articular surface. Buckwalter[10] has described

The authors did not receive grants or outside funding in the preparation of this manuscript. They did not receive payments or other benefits or a commitment or agreement to provide such benefits from a commercial entity. No commercial entity paid or directed, or agreed to pay or direct, any benefits to any research fund, foundation, educational institution, or other charitable or nonprofit organization with which the authors are affiliated or associated.

University of Kentucky Department of Orthopaedic Surgery and Sports Medicine, 740 S. Limestone, Suite K-408, Lexington, KY 40536-0284, USA
* Corresponding author.
E-mail address: clatt2@uky.edu (C. Lattermann).

Clin Sports Med 28 (2009) 285–301
doi:10.1016/j.csm.2008.10.007
0278-5919/08/$ – see front matter © 2009 Elsevier Inc. All rights reserved.

mechanisms of injury and subsequent response to injury in detail. Though perhaps a simplistic means summarizing years of research, the basic principle is such that partial-thickness tears (chondral fractures) do not heal and full-thickness tears (osteochondral fractures) heal variably, with a predominance of type I collagen with inferior biomechanical properties. A normal hyaline surface is not reproduced; instead, chondral lesions produce an irregular surface that predisposes the joint as well as soft-tissue structures to further injury.[11]

Unlike other forms of cartilage repair and restoration, osteochondral allografts take advantage of the inherently poor healing potential of articular cartilage in an attempt to restore a quasi-native joint surface. The goal is to replace what has been lost in a way that is as biologic and anatomic as possible. As articular cartilage is normally avascular, aneural, and alymphatic, newly transplanted chondrocytes are immersed in a familiar environment. Cells are embedded in an acellular matrix protecting them from host immunogenic cells.[12] Metabolic requirements continue to be met through the diffusion of synovial fluid.

Unfortunately, the subchondral component of the graft can be a source of difficulty if allograft tissue is not properly processed. The properties of subchondral bone differ tremendously from its overlying articular surface. Most importantly, transplanted bone is nonviable[13] and relies on the host for vascular invasion with subsequent osteoclastic resorption of dead bone and replacement with new viable bone (creeping substitution).[14] And along with the invading vessels into the newly transplanted bone come host immunogenic cells.

In essence, osteochondral allografts trade a severely damaged or absent articular surface for an intact one and replace viable with nonviable subchondral bone. The subchondral bone tends to heal, giving structural support to the overlying articular surface. As with osteochondral autografts, consistent healing of the chondral portion of the graft to the adjacent hyaline cartilage layer has not been shown.[10]

Although chondrocyte viability within osteochondral allografts has been documented by several studies,[15–17] the origin (host versus donor) of these cells within grafts could not be definitively confirmed despite several methods of analysis. Jamali and colleagues,[18] using fluorescence in situ hybridization (FISH) and karyotype analysis, recently reported conclusive evidence of donor-cell survival in a fresh osteochondral allograft at 29 years.

ADVANTAGES AND DISADVANTAGES OF OSTEOCHONDRAL ALLOGRAFTS

There are several structural, clinical, and theoretical advantages of osteochondral allografts over other types of articular cartilage restoration (autologous chondrocyte implantation, marrow stimulating techniques, and osteochondral autografts) (**Table 1**). First, a fully formed mature hyaline cartilage layer with viable chondrocytes capable

Table 1	
Advantages and disadvantages of osteochondral allografts	
Advantages	**Disadvantages**
Transplantation of mature hyaline cartilage	Potential for disease transmission
Restoration of joint contour	Potential for immunologic reaction
Relief of joint pain	Availability
Precise preparation of sizes	Demanding surgical technique
Lack of donor-site morbidity	

of maintaining the extracellular matrix is transplanted along with a variable-sized sub-chondral layer of bone.[15,19] No other method is capable of restoring large defects of subchondral bone as well as joint contour in a single operative procedure. Several studies have documented the ability of osteochondral allografts to be an effective means of replacing focal areas of damaged articular cartilage as well as relieving joint pain.[3,20,21] Although the relief of joint pain is not well understood, the current belief is centered on the replacement of innervated bone with denervated subchondral bone of the graft.

The clinical and surgical advantages of allografts have been well described: availability to the surgeon, precise preparation of graft material in any number of sizes, lack of donor-site morbidity, shorter operative times (one-stage operation) than other restorative procedures, and lack of clinically significant immunologic reactions.[22] In most cases, grafts may be harvested from a younger donor with healthier articular cartilage than that of the recipient.

Disadvantages include the potential for disease transmission, immunologic reaction with subsequent graft rejection, cost, limited availability of allografts, and demanding surgical technique. Increasing diagnostic technology as well as knowledge of treatment options has allowed the orthopedic surgeon the ability to offer cartilage restorative procedures that were not available in the past. The increasing demand of osteochondral allografts has, in essence, limited their availability.

PROCUREMENT AND STORAGE

The retrieval, processing, and allocation of allografts are highly monitored processes. The American Association of Tissue Banks (AATB) was founded in 1976 to establish standards and guidelines for procurement of allografts.[23] Initially, the use of fresh osteochondral allografts was limited to a small number of institutions in North America; however, in 1998, commercially supplied allografts became available in the United States. According to the AATB Web site (www.AATB.org), more than 100 accredited tissue banks are located in the United States today. All forms of bone allograft are primarily obtained from 3 sources: femoral head of a patient undergoing a total hip arthroplasty (THA), multi-organ donors, and postmortem donors. Allograft from a patient undergoing a THA is the most convenient because testing can be performed both pre- and postoperatively. Postmortem donors are most often rejected as retrieval often takes place in less-than-sterile environments despite sterile technique.[5]

Osteochondral allografts are stored as fresh, fresh-frozen, or cryopreserved grafts. Each of these storage options affects chondrocyte viability, immunogenicity, and length of time to transplantation. Fresh-frozen tissue that is maintained at $-80°C$ eliminates >95% of viable chondrocytes, because they are destroyed during the freezing process.[24] As chondrocytes are responsible for maintenance of the extracellular matrix, studies[25] have shown that the matrix in these frozen allografts tends to deteriorate over time. Deterioration of the matrix is evident by an increase in matrix metalloproteinases (MMPs), as reported by Acosta and colleagues.[26] Although decreased chondrocyte viability is not ideal, fresh-frozen allografts do exhibit decreased immunogenicity and, therefore, may be more appropriate for bulk allografting in major osseous reconstructions.[27]

Cryopreservation, on the other hand, is capable of maintaining chondrocyte viability during this freezing process by adding glycerol and dimethyl sulfoxide (DMSO) to the tissue. Theoretically, the addition of these chemicals prevents ice formation within cells and thus destruction of chondrocytes. Multiple studies[13,19,28–30] have reported variable results, with chondrocyte survival ranging from 20% to 70%. Unfortunately, cell survival appears to be limited to the surface of the articular cartilage layer.[31] Theories to explain this phenomenon include the inability to uniformly control the freezing rate of the tissue, disruption of cell membranes secondary to ice crystal formation, and inadequate penetration of glycerol or DMSO during the freezing. With the increase in tissue bank screening times and limited osteochondral allograft availability, research regarding cryopreservation will likely increase in the years to follow.

In multiple retrieval studies, fresh allografts have been shown to have the highest rates of chondrocyte viability of the 3 methods of storage[19,28,29,32] and are the most commonly used grafts in the United States. Fresh grafts are placed in lactated Ringer's solution or tissue culture medium at 4°C or 37°C, where they have historically been thought to be stored for 5 to 7 days before chondrocyte viability begins to decline. Fresh cold-stored osteochondral allografts have been shown to contain viable chondrocytes with maintenance of the extracellular matrix for many years after transplantation.[18,33,34] Ranawat and colleagues[35] reported superior histologic and biomechanical properties of cold-stored fresh allograft compared with freeze-thawed specimens. Gross and colleagues[36] recently examined histologic features of 35 fresh osteochondral allograft specimens and found that with a stable osseous graft base, the hyaline cartilage portion of the allograft could survive and function for 25 years or more. Research is ongoing to determine the most biologic means of reversing the metabolic suppression of cold-preserved grafts; gradual rewarming and decreasing nitric oxide at the time of graft implantation may have implications on graft survival.[37]

The length of time of storage before implantation has also been explored recently. Currently, fresh grafts are commercially available to clinicians approximately 14 to 21 days following graft harvest. Studies[38,39] have shown decreased chondrocyte viability and degradation of biomechanical properties of grafts stored for greater than 14 days. Malinin and colleagues[40] reported time-dependent loss of chondrocytes within cold-stored fresh allografts implanted into adult baboons, especially when stored for longer than 15 to 20 days. Williams and colleagues[41] recently revealed data showing that hypothermically stored fresh grafts implanted after a storage time of 17 to 42 days were effective at 2-year follow up. Grafts were determined to be effective both structurally and functionally in reconstructing symptomatic chondral and osteochondral lesions of the knee. Currently, the goal is to implant fresh osteochondral allografts as soon as possible, within 21 to 28 days of harvest.

RISK OF DISEASE TRANSMISSION

As with transplantation of any allogeneic tissue, viral and bacterial disease transmission is possible despite strenuous donor screening, aseptic technique, and testing of tissue.[42] Initial screening occurs long before tissue is retrieved by eliminating potential donors based on a full physical examination, immediate evidence of infection, and a review of the patient's relevant medical records after consent has been obtained. Aseptic technique is used during and after retrieval of tissues to limit contamination. In addition to testing for human immunodeficiency virus (HIV) types 1 and 2, hepatitis B virus (HBV), hepatitis C virus (HCV), and syphilis, the AATB requires testing for human T-cell lymphotropic virus (HTLV) I and II and uses nucleic acid testing (NAT) for HIV-1 and HCV, which is not yet required by the U.S. Food and Drug Administration (FDA). Polymerase chain reaction (PCR) testing is capable of decreasing the window of vulnerability from 4 to 6 weeks to approximately 10 days[43] in viruses known to have a "window" period, such as HIV and HCV.

Several methods of sterilization have been attempted, including low-dose gamma irradiation, antibiotic soaks, and a variety of inactivating agents (ethylene oxide, ether, and hydrogen peroxide). No perfect sterilization technique is currently available, because methods that completely eradicate viral and bacterial spores also disrupt collagen structure.[43] Currently, the most common method to ensure sterile grafts is sterile harvest and processing with low-dose (2.5 Mrad) gamma irradiation to kill surface pathogens.

Although the risks of acquiring disease through transplantation are very small, patients as well as surgeons remain concerned. Buck and colleagues[44] estimated the risk of HIV transmission in 1989 to be 1/1.6 million, though this estimate was before the advent of PCR testing. The last reported case of disease transmission from allograft tissue of all types was in 2002 (before NAT/PCR) when 40 patients received tissue from an anti-HCV-negative donor.[45] None of the 16 recipients receiving irradiated bone tested positive for HCV after transplantation. The only reported cases of tuberculosis and HBV in tissue recipients occurred more than 50 years ago. Interest arose in 2001 when a male recipient of allograft tissue expired secondary to an infection with Clostridium;[46] however, the tissue was retrieved by a facility that was not accredited by the AATB, and the donor's body had initially been refused by the local AATB-accredited tissue bank. According to the AATB in 2006, the majority of bacterial-contaminated transplants that have been reported in the literature have never been confirmed by the Centers for Disease Control and Prevention (CDC). Despite the relatively minuscule risks of disease transmission under today's standards, both the surgeon and patient should be aware of this possibility, and it must be discussed as a component of the informed-consent process.

IMMUNOGENICITY

Another important aspect of informed consent is the risk of immunologic reaction and/or rejection of the graft tissue. Small fragment allografts are not human leukocyte antigen (HLA)- or blood type-matched between the donor and recipient.[27] Host immune response to osteochondral allografts is elicited by the major histocompatibility complex (MHC) Class I and II antigens that are present on the surface of osteocytes and chondrocytes. Fortunately, an immune response against chondrocytes is limited secondary to the avascular and alymphatic cartilage matrix surrounding them. The cartilage matrix serves to shield the MHC Class I antigens from recognition by host cells, thereby protecting the chondrocytes from host immune response.[12]

In contrast to the articular cartilage layer of the graft, the osseous component of the graft expresses MHC cell-surface antigens, which come in contact with host immunogenic cells during vascular invasion and graft incorporation. In order to decrease the risk of this immune response, bone allograft is processed by multiple techniques (pulsatile irrigation, cold storage, and cytotoxic agents) to remove blood and bone marrow cells, thus creating a less immunogenic transplant.[42]

Although properly processed osteochondral allografts are relatively inert immunologically, showing little or no histologic evidence of an immune-mediated response,[14] Sirlin and colleagues[47] reported that 11 of 25 individuals generated serum anti-HLA antibodies after transplantation of shell allografts. Compared with antibody-negative patients, patients with anti-HLA antibodies showed an inferior appearance on magnetic resonance imaging (MRI). Statistically significant MRI findings of grafts in antibody-positive patients included greater mean edema, thicker interface, more abnormal marrow, and a higher proportion of surface collapse. The clinical significance of this finding is unknown, though further research is needed to determine the role of immune behavior in determining the outcome of fresh osteochondral allografts.[48]

INDICATIONS

Osteochondral allografts are primarily indicated for the treatment of full-thickness articular cartilage defects of 1 cm^2 or larger.[32,49,50] Although these types of defects are most often seen in young patients secondary to a traumatic event, other conditions that are amenable to osteochondral allografting include osteochondritis dissecans (OCD),[51,52] avascular necrosis,[53] as well as other conditions involving disease or absent underlying subchondral bone. Primary allograft can be considered for large lesions (>2 cm^2, 6–10 mm deep) less suited for other reparative or restorative procedures.[27] The degree of donor-site morbidity and limited availability of donor sites limit the use of autograft in these situations. Allografts have also been shown to be useful for salvage procedures after failure of other methods of cartilage repair and restoration, such as microfracture, autologous chondrocyte implantation, and mosaic-plasty.[54] Within the knee, osteochondral allografts have been used to treat posttraumatic and degenerative lesions associated with intra-articular tibial plateau fractures,[55,56] patellofemoral chondrosis or arthrosis,[57] and unicompartmental or multifocal osteoarthritis (**Fig. 1**).[58,59]

While the knee is by far the most common anatomic site for osteochondral allografting, other joints have also been treated with variable success.[60] Within the ankle, allografts have been used for resurfacing of the tibiotalar joint (bipolar) secondary to post-traumatic arthrosis,[61,62] osteonecrosis, and OCD lesions of the talus not amenable to other procedures, as well as reconstruction following excision of tumors of the calcaneus and talus.[63]

In 2001, Gross and colleagues[61] reported the results of osteochondral allografting performed in 9 patients with isolated osteochondral defects of the talar dome. Three of the 9 patients required eventual fusion secondary to resorption and fragmentation of the graft; however, the remaining 6 grafts remained in situ with a mean survival of 11 years, suggesting osteochondral allografts as viable options for focal defects of the talus. Jeng and colleagues[64] recently reported a 2-year follow-up of 29 patients

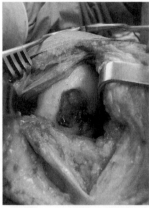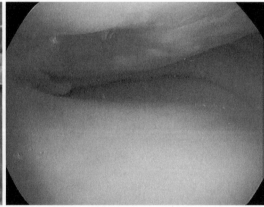

Fig. 1. Osteochondral defect in the knee. Osteochondral defects identified during open or arthroscopic surgery of the knee joint. Note the deep cavitation of the defects extending into and through the subchondral bone plate.

treated with bipolar osteochondral allografts of the tibiotalar joint performed for post-traumatic arthritis. Fourteen of the 29 patients required revision with the use of repeat ankle transplant, prosthetic total ankle arthroplasty, or bone block arthrodesis. Six of the remaining 15 transplants were deemed radiographic failures due to allograft fracture, allograft collapse, or progressive loss of joint space. The authors concluded that due to the extremely high failure rate, bipolar osteochondral allografting should only be considered in patients too young for ankle replacement, with excellent range of motion, low body mass index, normal radiographic alignment, and patients who refuse arthrodesis.

Although indications are less clear and few published data exist, osteochondral grafts have also been used with variable success in both the hip and shoulder joints. Indications include young patients with osteonecrosis of both the femoral head and humeral head[65,66] as well as large osteochondral lesions associated with glenohumeral dislocation and instability.[67]

CONTRAINDICATIONS

Understanding when the use of osteochondral allografts is not appropriate is critical during preoperative assessment. Operative candidates are chosen based on history, physical examination, and a thorough review of imaging studies. All of the following are essential portions of the preoperative assessment: age, activity level, and expectations of the patient; history of inflammatory arthropathies; location, size, and depth of defect; condition of surrounding articular cartilage; meniscal integrity; ligament instability; and limb alignment.[68]

Though allografting has been performed with some success in younger patients with multicompartmental arthrosis,[58,59] there is no role for osteochondral grafting in patients of appropriate age and activity level with progressive multicompartmental osteoarthritic changes.[27] These patients are best treated with primary prosthetic arthroplasty. Soft-tissue (meniscal, ligamentous) instability and malalignment of the limb must be addressed either concomitantly or at a separate procedure to provide the graft with an optimized environment for incorporation and function. Inflammatory disease (rheumatoid arthritis, crystal-induced arthropathy) and severe corticosteroid-induced osteonecrosis should be considered relative contraindications as well.[69] As mentioned earlier, all patients should understand the risks, benefits, and alternatives to the surgical procedure, with special interest focused on the potential for disease transmission and graft failure.

SURGICAL PLANNING

Although osteochondral allografts have been used in other joints, the majority of procedures and hence the literature have been documented regarding the knee; therefore, the following discussion on surgical technique is limited to the knee joint, specifically the femoral condyle.

Prior to performing any surgical procedure, a thorough preoperative plan with adequate radiographs must be formed. An important aspect of the preoperative plan is a thorough discussion with the patient regarding expectations of the procedure. Young active patients with focal chondral lesions secondary to trauma or OCD can be expected to return to normal activities after sufficient rehabilitation. Conversely, expectations for older individuals, often with chronic lesions, are often to delay the need for prosthetic replacement and reduce pain associated with functional activities of daily living.

As a part of the preoperative plan, many surgeons choose to perform a diagnostic knee arthroscopy before transplantation, verifying the soft-tissue status and overall quality of articular cartilage. Allografts are matched based on anterior-posterior radiographs of the knee, and the medial-lateral dimension of the tibia is measured just distal to the joint surface. After correction for magnification, this measurement is used by the tissue bank to match the donor tibial plateau. Other investigators[70] have used the affected condyle as a parameter for sizing. A match is considered acceptable based on size within ±2 mm, not taking into account variable anatomy, which may exist secondary to the pathologic or traumatic injury. For instance, the affected condyle in OCD is often larger, wider, and flatter, necessitating a large donor condyle.[27] Before beginning the operative procedure, the surgeon must thoroughly inspect the graft for appropriate sizing and quality of the tissue.

SURGICAL TECHNIQUE/GRAFT TECHNIQUES
Positioning/Access

The surgical technique for reconstruction of articular cartilage defects with osteochondral allografts has been described in detail by several authors.[27,32,60,71–73] The patient is positioned supine, a proximal thigh tourniquet is used, and maintenance of 70° to 100° of knee flexion is achieved with the use of a leg or foot holder. Transplantation generally requires an open procedure, typically performed through a midline approach while deviating subcutaneously either medially or laterally to the patellar tendon depending on the location of the lesion. A retinacular incision is then performed from proximal to distal to enter the joint, taking care not to damage the anterior horn of the meniscus or articular surface. Once the joint capsule and synovium have been incised, Z-retractors are placed medially or laterally as well as in the intercondylar notch to protect the cruciate ligaments. The knee is then taken through the range of motion to bring the defect into optimal view.

Once adequate access to the lesion is gained, a probe is used to palpate the size, depth, and quality of the margins of the defect (**Fig. 2**). After sizing is completed, a punch is used to delineate the diameter of the graft needed. A dowel-type drill is used to ream a precise socket down to the level of healthy subchondral bone, indicated by punctate hemorrhage. In focal chondral defects, this depth should be approximately 8 mm; however, in lesions secondary to OCD, the depth may be substantially larger (**Fig. 3**). Lesions involving the tibial plateau or the patella may require a more extensive resection as well.[74] If the depth of the lesion is extensive, morselized autologous bone graft should be used to fill the osseous defect. After the size, shape, and depth of the prepared bed is determined, the graft is ready for insertion.

Dowel (Press-Fit) Allografts

Depending on the location and size of the lesion, 2 techniques (dowel, shell) can be used in preparation and implantation of osteochondral allografts. Dowel allograft, the more commonly used technique, involves inserting either a single precisely contoured plug or multiple plugs placed closely together at various angles to match the curvature of the lesion to be resurfaced. A single press-fit plug is optimal, as space between multiple plugs is subject to the formation of fibrocartilage with uneven cobblestoning, which may affect clinical outcome.[60]

Dowel allografts are usually 8 mm thick in focal chondral defects and up to 15 mm thick in OCD lesions. They are primarily recommended for condylar lesions between 15 and 35 mm in diameter. Unlike shell autografts, press-fit grafts generally do not require additional fixation; however, careful insertion of the graft by dilating the recipient

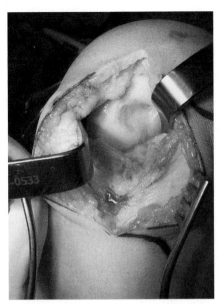

Fig. 2. Partially uncontained defect after failed repair of osteochondritis dissecans (OCD). Particularly in a revision situation after previously failed surgery, it is critical to evaluate the location of the defect. In patients with failed OCD lesions, the defect is often partially uncontained, and the shape of the condyle can be significantly altered. The use of a full hemicondyle graft is, therefore, recommended to be able to ideally match the graft to the defect.

site with a slightly oversized tamp must be achieved to prevent excessive impact loading of the articular surface. Borazjani and colleagues[75] reported that chondrocyte death, particularly in the superficial zone, occurred during impact insertion of dowel grafts and recommended further research regarding insertion techniques.

Technical difficulty with the use of the circular coring system limits the use of the dowel technique in certain locations, such as the posterior femur, tibia, patella, and trochlea. The use of circular plugs may also require extensive removal of normal adjacent cartilage to achieve a stable fit.

Shell Allografts

Shell allografts define the "art" of osteochondral allografting. Using freehand technique, grafts are matched to the outlined defect, minimizing sacrifice of normal articular cartilage. The graft is initially oversized followed by meticulous sculpting to achieve an exact fit. Bioabsorbable pins or low-profile interfragmentary screws are often needed for fixation. The most obvious disadvantage is the technically demanding nature of the procedure, limiting its use by many surgeons. Primary indications for shell allografts include larger lesions with an asymmetric pattern located in regions not amenable to dowel allografts.

Technical Considerations

Whether using the dowel or shell technique, several generalized aspects of the procedure are worthy of special attention. Matching the radius of curvature of the graft to host anatomy is critical to avoid increased contact pressure and restoring joint contour, especially with shell autografts (**Fig. 4**).[76] Before insertion, allografts are

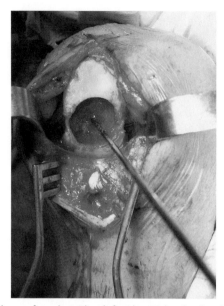

Fig. 3. Preparation of the graft socket. The defect has to be sized such that the entire defect can be cut out with a circular reamer. The graft socket is prepared deep enough to reach bleeding bone. Ideally, this should be 8 mm deep, but in a failed OCD lesion, it is necessary to reach bleeding subchondral bone. This may require a socket that can be up to 10 or 15 mm deep.

subjected to pulsatile lavage to remove blood and bone marrow cells in a final attempt to decrease the risk of a host immune response.[77] The final resting position of the graft relative to the surrounding articular surface has been controversial. Initially, many authors believed that by placing the graft 1 mm proud, the graft would eventually become flush with adjacent tissue after subsidence and resorption occurred in the weeks to follow.[16,78] Studies exploring contact pressures within grafts[79,80] have questioned leaving the graft proud by demonstrating that the level of the graft can have a tremendous effect on contact pressures within the graft. Grafts elevated 0.5 to

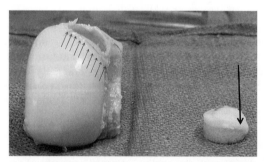

Fig. 4. Preparation of the allograft. During the preparation of the allograft, it is important to do a precise match with the recipient condyle. Particularly in partially uncontained defects, it is important to match the curvature (*black arrows*) well to the recipient to avoid recessing the graft.

1.0 mm appeared to have up to a 50% increase in contact pressure. Conversely, grafts that were flush or even slightly recessed restored normal contact pressures (**Fig. 5**).

Postoperative Management

Postoperative management is similar to other cartilage reparative and restorative procedures focusing on weight-bearing protection and regaining joint range of motion. Unless other concomitant procedures (meniscal repair, ligament reconstruction, or osteotomy) are performed at the time of transplantation, early full range of motion is encouraged to prevent adhesions.

Postoperative rehabilitation is divided into 4 phases. During phase I (0–6 weeks), the patient is made non-weight bearing on the affected extremity, and a continuous passive motion (CPM) device is used for 6 to 8 hours per day. Range of motion is initially limited to 0° to 40°, increasing 5° to 10° per day as patient comfort allows. The patient should gain 100° by week 6. A total-range-of-motion (TROM) brace is used, initially locked in extension for the first postoperative week and removed only for CPM and exercises. During weeks 2 to 4, the brace is gradually opened in 20° increments as quadriceps control is gained. Bracing is discontinued when a straight-leg raise can be controlled without an extension lag. Exercises during phase I include passive and active-assisted knee range of motion to tolerance as well as stretching and strengthening of the quadriceps, hamstrings, and gluteus muscles.

During phase II (6–8 weeks), partial weight-bearing (25%) is allowed, and knee flexion to 130° should be achieved. Stretching and strengthening exercises are continued with the addition of a stationary bike to improve range of motion. Phase III (8–12 weeks) allows gradual return to full weight bearing, with progression to full, pain-free, knee range of motion. Gait training and closed-chain exercises (wall sits, shuttle, mini-squats, and toe raise) are performed. Phase IV (12 weeks–6 months) concludes

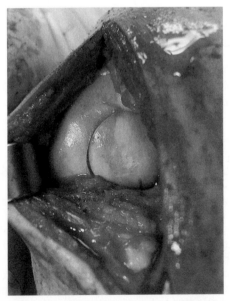

Fig. 5. Implantation of fresh osteochondral allograft to the femoral condyle. A near-perfect restoration of the curvature of the condyle as well as very tight limits on the recess of the graft is critical for the clinical outcome.

with a full and normalized gait pattern associated with full and pain-free knee range of motion. Return to activities is allowed between 6 to 12 months depending on progression.

Other authors[27,48] have recommended slightly different postoperative protocols. Key differences include immediate toe-touch weight bearing for 6 to 8 weeks, or longer, depending on the size of the graft, type of fixation, and radiographic evidence of graft incorporation. Closed-chain kinetic chain exercises, such as cycling, are often started at 4 weeks postoperatively. Unrestricted low-demand activities are usually allowed by 3 to 4 months. Braces are often not recommended during rehabilitation, except in the case of patellofemoral grafts, which need early protection by limiting knee flexion to <45° for the first 4 to 6 weeks.

Results

Clinical results of fresh osteochondral allografts used in the treatment of focal osteochondral defects of the knee have shown encouraging long-term results.[32,34,41,51,53,55,56,59,71,73,81] Overall success rates have been reported ranging from 10% to 95%, with etiologies that include posttraumatic lesions, osteonecrosis, and OCD. An extensive review of results has been performed recently.[27,60] Gross and colleagues[34] found that performing concomitant procedures at the time of osteochondral transplantation had no significant difference with respect to outcome rating or rates of failure. Multiple studies have shown less favorable results with osteochondral allograft use in bipolar reconstruction of the femur and tibia[32,55,71] as well as the patellofemoral joint.[57,71] Spak and colleagues[82] retrospectively reviewed 14 patients younger than 55 years of age treated with fresh osteochondral allografts for patellofemoral arthritis. At an average of 10 years' follow-up, 8 grafts were in place, 4 for more than 10 years and 2 for more than 5 years. Of the nonsurviving allografts, 3 had survived more than 10 years. Radiographs showed intact allografts with mild or no degenerative changes. Average Knee Society scores also improved, prompting the authors to challenge previous results regarding patellofemoral allografting.

Several studies regarding survivorship of grafts have recently been reported. Gross and colleagues[36] examined histologic features of 35 fresh osteochondral allograft specimens retrieved at the time of subsequent graft revision, osteotomy, or total knee arthroplasty. Given chondrocyte viability, long-term allograft survival appeared to depend on the stability of host-graft bone interface. In 2007, Jamali and colleagues[18] and Maury and colleagues[83] reported chondrocyte stability at 29 and 25 years, respectively.

COMPLICATIONS

Fortunately, complications such as disease transmission, infection, and immunogenic reaction are rare. Superficial and deep infections must be distinguished on the basis of laboratory markers, physical examination, and joint aspiration. Deep infections necessitate removal of the graft.

Allograft failure may occur both early and late after transplantation. Early failure occurs as a result of chondrocyte death and may be a function of the length and type of storage before transplantation.[40] Late failures show fracture of the graft, incomplete remodeling of the graft-bone interface, and resorption of the graft tissue by synovial activity at the graft edge.[36] Graft fragmentation and collapse typically occur in areas of the subchondral bone noted to have limited revascularization. Patients with graft failure often present with new-onset pain or mechanical symptoms.[27] MRI may be helpful in ruling out other etiologies of postoperative symptoms; however, caution must be exercised, because normally functioning grafts may also exhibit signal abnormalities. Progression of the disease process or infection may also be the origin of new-onset pain and mechanical symptoms, causing diagnostic confusion. Treatment options for graft failure include observation, bracing, removal of the graft with or without repeat allografting, or conversion to arthroplasty.

SUMMARY

The treatment of osteochondral defects continues to be a difficult problem for both patients and clinicians. As with all treatment options, patients should be made aware of the potential risks and complications associated with the use of osteochondral allografts. Although research and techniques for repair and restoration of articular cartilage continue to develop, osteochondral allografting is currently the only technique capable of restoring mature hyaline cartilage.

REFERENCES

1. Bolano L, Kopta JA. The immunology of bone and cartilage transplantation. Orthopedics 1991;14:987–96.
2. Lexer E. Joint transplantations and arthroplasty. Surg Gynecol Obstet 1925;40: 782–809.
3. Meyers MH, Akeson W, Convery FR. Resurfacing of the knee with fresh osteochondral allograft. J Bone Joint Surg Am 1989;71:704–13.
4. Greenwald S, Boden S, Goldberg V, et al. Bone-graft substitutes: facts, fictions, and applications. J Bone Joint Surg Am 2001;83(Suppl 2):98–103.
5. Delloye C, Cornu O, Druez V, et al. Bone allografts: what they can offer and what they cannot. J Bone Joint Surg Br 2007;89:574–80.
6. Brittberg M, Lindahl A, Nilsson A, et al. Treatment of deep cartilage defects in the knee with autologous chondrocyte transplantation. N Engl J Med 1994;331: 889–95.
7. Hangody L, Fules P. Autologous osteochondral mosaicplasty for the treatment of full-thickness defects of weight-bearing joints: ten years of experimental and clinical experience. J Bone Joint Surg Am 2003;85(Suppl 2):25–32.
8. Hubbard MJ. Arthroscopic surgery for chondral flaps in the knee. J Bone Joint Surg Br 1987;69:794–6.
9. Steadman JR, Briggs KK, Rodrigo JJ, et al. Outcomes of microfracture for traumatic chondral defects of the knee: average 11-year follow-up. Arthroscopy 2003;19:477–84.
10. Buckwalter JA. Articular cartilage injuries. Clin Orthop Relat Res 2002;402:21–37.
11. Hjelle K, Solheim E, Strand T, et al. Articular cartilage defects in 1,000 knee arthroscopies. Arthroscopy 2002;18:730–4.
12. Langer F, Gross AE. Immunogenicity of allograft articular cartilage. J Bone Joint Surg Am 1974;56:297–304.
13. Rodrigo JJ, Thompson E, Travis C. Deep-freezing versus 4 degrees preservation of avascular osteocartilaginous shell allografts in rats. Clin Orthop Relat Res 1987;218:268–75.
14. Oakeshott RD, Farine I, Pritzker KP, et al. A clinical and histological analysis of failed fresh osteochondral allografts. Clin Orthop Relat Res 1988;233:283–94.
15. Czitrom AA, Keating S, Gross AE. The viability of articular cartilage in fresh osteochondral allografts after clinical transplantation. J Bone Joint Surg Am 1990;72: 574–81.

16. Convery FR, Akeson WH, Amiel D, et al. Long-term survival of chondrocytes in an osteochondral articular cartilage allograft. A case report. J Bone Joint Surg Am 1996;78:1082–8.
17. McGoveran BM, Pritzker KP, Shasha N, et al. Long-term chondrocytes viability in a fresh osteochondral allograft. J Knee Surg 2002;15:97–100.
18. Jamali AA, Hatcher SL, You Z. Donor cell survival in a fresh osteochondral allograft at twenty-nine years. A case report. J Bone Joint Surg Am 2007;89(1): 166–9.
19. Schachar N, McAllister D, Stevenson M, et al. Metabolic and biochemical status of articular cartilage following cryopreservation and transplantation: A rabbit model. J Orthop Res 1992;10:603–9.
20. Bobic V. Arthroscopic osteochondral autograft transplantation in anterior cruciate ligament reconstruction: a preliminary clinical study. Knee Surg Sports Traumatol Arthrosc 1996;3:262–4.
21. McDermott AG, Langer F, Pritzker KP, et al. Fresh small-fragment osteochondral allografts: long term follow-up study on first 100 cases. Clin Orthop 1985;197: 96–102.
22. Harner CD, Olson E, Irrgang JJ, et al. Allograft versus autograft anterior cruciate ligament reconstruction: 3- to 5-year outcome. Clin Orthop 1996;324: 134–44.
23. American Association of Tissue Banks. Standards for tissue banking. Arlington (VA): American Association of Tissue Banks; 1987.
24. Enneking WF, Mindell ER. Observations on massive retrieved human allografts. J Bone Joint Surg Am 1991;73:1123–42.
25. Enneking WF, Campanacci DA. Retrieved human allografts: a clinicopathological study. J Bone Joint Surg Am 2001;83:971–86.
26. Acosta CA, Izal I, Ripalda P, et al. Cell viability and protein composition in cryopreserved cartilage. Clin Orthop Relat Res 2007;460:234–9.
27. Görtz S, Bugbee WD. Allografts in articular cartilage repair. Instr Course Lect 2007;56:469–80.
28. Conway B, Tomford W, Mankin HJ, et al. Radiosensitivity of HIV-1: potential application to sterilization of bone allografts. AIDS 1991;5:608–9.
29. Malinin TI, Wagner JL, Pita JC, et al. Hypothermic storage and cryopreservation of cartilage. Clin Orthop 1985;187:15–26.
30. Tomford WW, Duff GP, Mankin HJ. Experimental freeze preservation of chondrocytes. Clin Orthop 1985;197:11–4.
31. Judas F, Rosa S, Teixeira L, et al. Chondrocyte viability in fresh and frozen large human osteochondral allografts: effect of cryoprotective agents. Transplant Proc 2007;39(8):2531–4.
32. Bugbee WD, Convery RF. Osteochondral allograft transplantation. Clin Sports Med 1999;18:67–75.
33. Sammarco VJ, Gorab R, Miller R, et al. Human articular cartilage storage in cell culture medium: guidelines for storage of fresh osteochondral allografts. Orthopedics 1997;20:497–500.
34. Gross AE, Shasha N, Aubin P. Long-term follow-up of the use of fresh osteochondral allografts for posttraumatic knee defects. Clin Orthop Relat Res 2005;435: 79–87.
35. Ranawat AS, Vidal AF, Chen CT, et al. Material properties of fresh cold-stored allografts for osteochondral defects at 1 year. Clin Orthop Relat Res 2008;466(8): 1826–36.

36. Gross AE, Kim W, Las Heras F, et al. Fresh osteochondral allografts for posttraumatic knee defects: long-term follow-up. Clin Orthop Relat Res 2008;466(8): 1863–70.
37. Pylawka TK, Virdi AS, Cole BJ, et al. Reversal of suppressed metabolism in prolonged cold preserved cartilage. J Orthop Res 2008;26(2):247–54.
38. Ball ST, Amiel D, Williams SK, et al. The effects of storage on fresh human osteochondral allografts. Clin Orthop Relat Res 2004;418:246–52.
39. Pearsall AW IV, Tucker JA, Hester RB, et al. Chondrocyte viability in refrigerated osteochondral allografts used for transplantation within the knee. Am J Sports Med 2004;32:125–31.
40. Malinin T, Temple HT, Buck BE. Transplantation of osteochondral allografts after cold storage. J Bone Joint Surg Am 2006;88(4):762–70.
41. Williams RJ III, Ranawat AS, Potter HG, et al. Fresh stored allografts for the treatment of osteochondral defects of the knee. J Bone Joint Surg Am 2007;89(4): 718–26.
42. Tomford WW. Transmission of disease through transplantation of musculoskeletal allografts. J Bone Joint Surg Am 1995;77:1742–54.
43. Caldwell PE III, Shelton WR. Indications for allografts. Orthop Clin North Am 2005; 36(4):459–67.
44. Buck BE, Malinin TI, Brown MD. Bone transplantation and human immunodeficiency virus: an estimate of risk of acquired immunodeficiency syndrome (AIDS). Clin Orthop 1989;240:129–36.
45. Tugwell BD, Patel PR, Williams IT, et al. Transmission of hepatitis C virus to several organ and tissue recipients from an antibody-negative donor. Ann Intern Med 2005;143(9):648–54.
46. Centers for Disease Control and Prevention. Update: allograft associated bacterial infections—United States, 2002. MMWR Morb Mortal Wkly Rep 2002;51: 207–10.
47. Sirlin CB, Brossmann J, Boutin RD, et al. Shell osteochondral allografts of the knee: comparison of MR imaging findings and immunologic responses. Radiology 2001;219:35–43.
48. Phipatanakul WP, VandeVord PJ, Teitge RA, et al. Immune response in patients receiving fresh osteochondral allografts. Am J Orthop 2004;33:345–8.
49. Lewis PB, McCarty LP III, Kang RW, et al. Basic science and treatment options for articular cartilage injuries. J Orthop Sports Phys Ther 2006;36(10):717–27.
50. Lattermann CL, Kang RW, Cole BJ. What's new in the treatment of focal chondral defects of the knee? Orthopedics 2006;29(10):898–903.
51. Garrett JC. Fresh osteochondral allografts for treatment of articular defects in osteochondritis dissecans of the lateral femoral condyle in adults. Clin Orthop 1994; 303:33–7.
52. Emmerson BC, Görtz S, Jamali AA, et al. Fresh osteochondral allografting in the treatment of osteochondritis dissecans of the femoral condyle. Am J Sports Med 2007;35(6):907–14.
53. Flynn JM, Springfield DS, Mankin HJ. Osteoarticular allografts to treat distal femoral osteonecrosis. Clin Orthop 1994;303:38–43.
54. Browne JE, Branch TP. Surgical alternatives for treatment of articular cartilage lesions. J Am Acad Orthop Surg 2000;8:180–9.
55. Ghazavi MT, Pritzker KP, Davis AM, et al. Fresh osteochondral allografts for posttraumatic osteochondral defects of the knee. J Bone Joint Surg Br 1997;79: 1008–13.

56. Shasha N, Krywulak S, Backstein D. Long-term follow-up of fresh tibial osteo-chondral allografts for failed tibial plateau fractures. J Bone Joint Surg Am 2003;85(Suppl 2):33–9.
57. Jamali AA, Emmerson BC, Chung C, et al. Fresh osteochondral allografts: results in the patellofemoral joint. Clin Orthop Relat Res 2005;437:176–85.
58. Gross AE, Silverstein EA, Falk J, et al. The allotransplantation of partial joints in the treatment of osteoarthritis of the knee. Clin Orthop Relat Res 1975;108: 7–14.
59. Beaver RJ, Mahomed M, Backstein D, et al. Fresh osteochondral allografts for post-traumatic defects in the knee. A survivorship analysis. J Bone Joint Surg Br 1992;74:105–10.
60. Hennig A, Abate J. Osteochondral allografts in the treatment of articular cartilage injuries of the knee. Sports Med Arthrosc 2007;15(3):126–32.
61. Gross AE, Agnidis Z, Hutchison CR. Osteochondral defects of the talus treated with fresh osteochondral allograft transplantation. Foot Ankle Int 2001;22:385–91.
62. Meehan R, McFarlin S, Bugbee W, et al. Fresh ankle osteochondral allograft transplantation for tibiotalar joint arthritis. Foot Ankle Int 2005;26:793–802.
63. Schoenfeld AJ, Leeson MC, Grossman JP. Fresh-frozen osteochondral allograft reconstruction of a giant cell tumor of the talus. J Foot Ankle Surg 2007;46(3): 144–8.
64. Jeng CL, Kadakia A, White KL, et al. Fresh osteochondral total ankle allograft transplantation for the treatment of ankle arthritis. Foot Ankle Int 2008;29(6): 554–60.
65. Meyers MH. Resurfacing of the femoral head with fresh osteochondral allografts. Long-term results. Clin Orthop Relat Res 1985;197:111–4.
66. Johnson DL, Warner JJ. Osteochondritis dissecans of the humeral head: treat-ment with a matched osteochondral allograft. J Shoulder Elbow Surg 1997;6: 160–3.
67. Chapovsky F, Kelly JD IV. Osteochondral allograft transplantation for treatment of glenohumeral instability. Arthroscopy 2005;21:1007.
68. Sgaglione N, Miniaci A, Gillogly S, et al. Update on advanced surgical techniques in the treatment of traumatic focal articular cartilage lesions in the knee. Arthros-copy 2002;18:9–32.
69. Shelton WR, Treacy SH, Dukes AD, et al. Use of allografts in knee reconstruction II: surgical considerations. J Am Acad Orthop Surg 1998;6:169–75.
70. Highgenboten CL, Jackson A, Trudelle-Jackson E, et al. Cross-validation of height and gender estimations of femoral condyle width in osteochondral allo-grafts. Clin Orthop Relat Res 1994;298:246–9.
71. Chu CR, Convery RF, Akeson WH, et al. Articular cartilage transplantation: clinical results in the knee. Clin Orthop 1999;360:159–68.
72. Garrett JC. Osteochondral allografts for reconstruction of articular defects of the knee. In: Cannon WD Jr, editor. Instructional course lectures 47. Rosemont (IL): American Academy of Orthopaedic Surgeons; 1998. p. 517–22.
73. Zukor D, Gross A. Osteochondral allograft reconstruction of the knee. Am J Knee Surg 1989;2:139–49.
74. Gortz S, Bugbee W. Fresh osteochondral allografts: graft processing and clinical applications. J Knee Surg 2006;19:231–9.
75. Borazjani BH, Chen AC, Bae WC, et al. Effect of impact on chondrocyte viability during insertion of human osteochondral grafts. J Bone Joint Surg Am 2006; 88(9):1934–43.

76. Tom JA, Rodeo SA. Soft tissue allografts for knee reconstruction in sports medicine. Clin Orthop 2002;402:135–56.
77. Lewandrowski KU, Rebmann V, Passler M, et al. Immune response to perforated and partially demineralized bone allografts. J Orthop Sci 2001;6:545–55.
78. Cooper JL, Beck CL. History of soft tissue allograft in orthopaedics. Sports Medicine & Arthoscopy Review 1993;1(1):2–16.
79. Koh JL, Wirsing K, Lautenschlager E, et al. The effect of graft height mismatch on contact pressure following osteochondral grafting: a biomechanical model. Am J Sports Med 2004;32:317–20.
80. Koh JL, Kowalski A, Lautenschlager E. The effect of angled osteochondral grafting on contact pressure: a biomechanical study. Am J Sports Med 2006;34: 116–9.
81. McCulloch PC, Kang RW, Sobhy MH, et al. Prospective evaluation of prolonged fresh osteochondral allograft transplantation of the femoral condyle: minimum 2-year follow-up. Am J Sports Med 2007;35:411–20.
82. Spak RT, Teitge RA. Fresh osteochondral allografts for patellofemoral arthritis: long-term follow-up. Clin Orthop Relat Res 2006;444:193–200.
83. Maury AC, Safir O, Heras FL, et al. Twenty-five-year chondrocyte viability in fresh osteochondral allograft. A case report. J Bone Joint Surg Am 2007;89(1):159–65.

Collateral Ligament Augmentation versus Reconstruction Using Allograft Tissue

Walter R. Shelton, MD

KEYWORDS

• MCL • LCL • Allograft • Popliteus combined instability

MEDIAL COLLATERAL LIGAMENT

The medial collateral ligament (MCL) is a broad strong ligament originating from the medial epicondyle of the femur (**Fig. 1**). It runs distally for approximately 10 to 12 cm and inserts on the medial tibial metaphysis 4 cm below the joint line. The MCL is the primary static stabilizer against valgus stress of the knee.

Tears of the MCL are the most common knee ligament injury. They are graded as grade I, when ligament fibers are torn but not completely disrupted and there is no instability. In grade II tears, the fibers are partially torn allowing for up to 5 mm of pathologic joint opening, but the ligament is intact enough to offer resistance against complete opening of the joint. In grade III tears, the ligament is completely disrupted and offers no restraint to valgus opening of the knee joint.

Isolated MCL tears are usually treated nonoperatively regardless of the grade of the tear. Woo and colleagues[1] showed in a dog model that the MCL healed without primary repair. Early range of motion with protection against recurrent valgus stress allows the ligament to heal with resulting good stability in almost all cases.[2] When the MCL is torn in combination with either the anterior cruciate ligament (ACL) or the posterior cruciate ligament (PCL), the resulting instability is much more complex and disabling. Hughston[3] felt that the MCL and ACL act synergistically in knee stability, especially as the knee approaches full extension. With acute tears, open repair has been advocated at the time of ACL reconstruction, and Marshall[4] felt this produced the most stable knee. Shelbourne,[5] however, has advocated reconstruction of the ACL with conservative treatment of the MCL to lessen the danger of arthrofibrosis associated with open MCL repair. Most surgeons prefer to treat the MCL conservatively when in combination with a cruciate ligament injury and reconstruct the ACL or PCL.

Mississippi Sports Medicine and Orthopaedic Center, 1325 East Fortification Street, Jackson, MS 39202, USA
E-mail address: wsheltonmd@msmoc.com

Clin Sports Med 28 (2009) 303–310
doi:10.1016/j.csm.2008.10.012
0278-5919/08/$ – see front matter © 2009 Elsevier Inc. All rights reserved.

sportsmed.theclinics.com

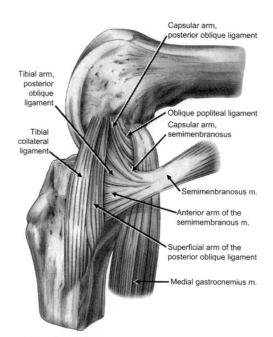

Capsular arm, posterior oblique ligament

Tibial arm, posterior oblique ligament

Tibial collateral ligament

Oblique popliteal ligament

Capsular arm, semimenbranosus

Semimenbranosus m.

Anterior arm of the semimembranous m.

Superficial arm of the posterior oblique ligament

Medial gastrocnemius m.

Fig.1. Medial collateral ligament. (*From* Johnson DH, Johnson P, Alsuwaidi A. Basic science of the knee. In: Johnson DH, Pedowitz RA, editors. Practical orthopaedic sports medicine and arthroscopy. Philadelphia: Lippincott, Williams and Wilkins; 2006; with permission.)

    Chronic MCL instability can be a difficult problem to address, especially when in combination with chronic ACL or PCL instability. When correcting chronic combined medial/cruciate instability, the cruciate ligament must be reconstructed at the time of reconstruction of the MCL. Secondary repair of the MCL by advancement of the ligament and augmentation with a tendon autograft, such as the semitendinosus, has been advocated as a way to overcome chronic combined MCL instability. The semitendinosus has been used both with a distal based attachment and attachment to the medial epicondyle through a drill hole and by attaching both proximal and distal ends through drill holes with a free graft.[6–8] Hughston and Andrews[9] advocated reinforcing the medial structures with a tightening of the posterior oblique ligament. Allograft reconstruction of the MCL involves tissue augmentation of the ligament with attachment through drill holes both at the tibial and femoral insertion sites. Wahl and Nicandri[10] advocate using the Achilles tendon allograft to reconstruct both the PCL and the MCL with 1 graft (**Fig. 2**). Borden and colleagues[11] advocated reconstructing the MCL with a double-bundle allograft using an anterior tibialis tendon allograft forming the anterior and posterior bundle for the MCL (**Fig. 4**). Shino and colleagues[7] reconstruct the MCL with a bone-patellar tendon-bone (BPTB) graft securing the bone plug in tunnels at the bony attachments of the MCL (**Fig. 3**). Excellent stability was achieved at 1 year using this technique in a canine model. Rehabilitation of a reconstructed or augmented MCL repair should include early, protected, full range of motion. The reconstructed ligament should be isometric, and early motion is desirable to prevent the complication of arthrofibrosis, especially in combined reconstruction of either the ACL or PCL. The MCL augmentation or reconstruction can be protected with a brace that allows for early weight bearing and protected motion.

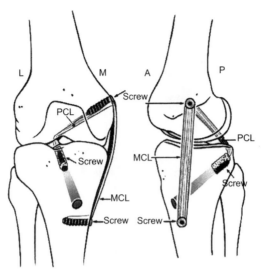

Fig. 2. Achilles allograft reconstruction of MCL and PCL. (*From* Wahl CJ, Nicandri G. Single-Achilles allograft posterior cruciate ligament and medial collateral ligament reconstruction: a technique to avoid osseous tunnel intersection, improve construct stiffness, and save on allograft utilization. Arthroscopy 2008;24:487; with permission.)

LATERAL COLLATERAL LIGAMENT AND POSTEROLATERAL CORNER

The lateral collateral ligament (LCL) originates from the lateral femoral epicondyle and inserts on the fibular head with an overall length of approximately 60 to 65 mm. It is the primary static stabilizer against varus stress of the knee. Along with the popliteus tendon and the popliteofibular ligament, the LCL also functions to provide rotational stability for the posterolateral corner (**Fig. 4**). The LCL and posterolateral structures are often injured in combination with either a PCL or ACL tear.

Acute tears of the LCL and posterolateral corner can cause disabling instability. The loss of the lateral meniscus increases rotational instability due to the loss of its bumper effect and the more convex shape of the lateral tibial plateau as compared with the medial tibial plateau. Acute tears of the LCL are grade I when the ligament has

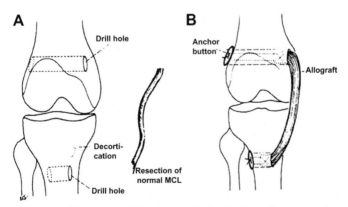

Fig. 3. Reconstruction of MCL using BPTB. (*From* Horibe A, Shino K, Nagano J, et al. Replacing the medial collateral ligament with an allogeneic tendon graft: an experimental canine study. J Bone Joint Surg Br 1990;72B:1044–9; with permission.)

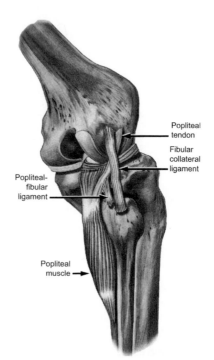

Poppliteal
tendon

Fibular
collateral
ligament

Poppliteal-
fibular
ligament

Poppliteal
muscle ➤

Fig. 4. Lateral collateral ligament. (*From* Johnson DH, Johnson P, Alsuwaidi A. Basic science of the knee. In: Johnson DH, Pedowitz RA, editors. Practical orthopaedic sports medicine and arthroscopy. Philadelphia: Lippincott, Williams and Wilkins; 2006; with permission.)

interstitial damage but there is no instability present. Grade II occurs when the ligament has 3 to 5 mm of laxity but remains in continuity. Grade III tears involve complete disruption of the LCL. In all LCL injuries with instability, primary repair should be considered, especially when combined with posterolateral corner and cruciate ligament injuries. Conservative treatment is recommended only for grade I tears with no clinical patholaxity.

Open primary repair of an acute grade II or grade III lateral collateral and posterolateral corner injury requires direct repair of torn structures and augmentation with either autograft or allograft tissue. The most common tissue used in augmenting the LCL is a strip of biceps femoris tendon or iliotibial band that is left attached distally and fixed to the femoral epicondyle through a small drill hole.

Isolated LCL is rare but has been described by Coobs and LaPrade.[12] They advocate primarily reconstructing the LCL using an autogenous semitendinosus graft. Any soft tissue allograft, including semitendinosus, anterior tibialis, or posterior tibialis, is an excellent choice to augment the acute repair of an LCL.

Chronic LCL and posterolateral instability is often associated with tears of the ACL or PCL. Conservative treatment for this instability is not usually successful, and reconstructive surgery of both the cruciate injury and lateral and posterolateral corner is necessary. Surgical reconstruction for this combined instability can be extremely challenging. Limb alignment is crucial to the success of any ligament reconstruction. If the leg is in varus alignment, a valgus osteotomy is always recommended as the initial procedure. Ligament reconstruction of the lateral and posterior lateral ligaments in a varus knee is doomed to failure.

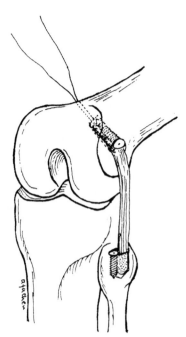

Fig. 5. LCL Reconstruction with quadriceps graft. (*From* Chen CH, Chen WJ, Shih CH. Lateral collateral ligament reconstruction using quadriceps tendon-patellar bone autograft with bioscrew fixation. Arthroscopy 2001;17:553; with permission.)

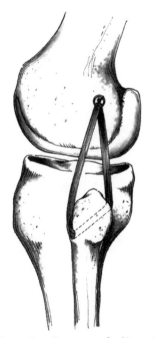

Fig. 6. LCL Reconstruction with semitendinosus graft. (*From* Kocabey Y, Nawab A, Caborn DNM, et al. Posterolateral corner reconstruction using a hamstring allograft and a bioabsorbable tenodesis screw: description of a new surgical technique. Arthroscopy 2004;20:162; with permission.)

Ligament reconstruction is advocated once the osteotomy is healed. If the lateral meniscus has been removed, replacement with a meniscus allograft transplant should be considered. The absence of a meniscus and persistent cruciate instability will contribute to the failure of lateral side reconstruction.

Numerous reconstruction techniques using both autogenous tissue and allograft tissue have been described to reconstruct the lateral corner. Latimer and colleagues[13] and Noyes and colleagues[14] have described reconstructing the LCL with a BPTB allograft. Both report a high degree of success controlling varus laxity and excessive external tibial rotation. Chin[15] has described using a quadriceps tendon graft with a bone plug to reconstruct the LCL (**Fig. 5**).

Other reconstructive techniques have centered on reconstructing both the popliteal fibular ligament and the popliteus tendon in combination with the LCL. A soft tissue graft with adequate length is necessary to achieve this reconstruction. Müller[16] described reconstructing an LCL, the popliteus tendon, and the popliteal fibular ligament with drill holes from the femur, tibia, and fibula according to the anatomic insertion of each structure. A drawback to these reconstructions is the replacement of a dynamic stabilizer, the popliteus tendon, with a static tendon graft. Markolf and colleagues[17] and Nau and colleagues[18] have shown excellent stability with reconstructing all 3 structures. Larson described reconstructing the LCL and popliteus with a figure-of-eight weave using a semitendinosus tendon.[19] Kocabey and Kaborn[20] and Arciero[21] and Kim[22] have all reported good stability with similar reconstruction of the LCL and

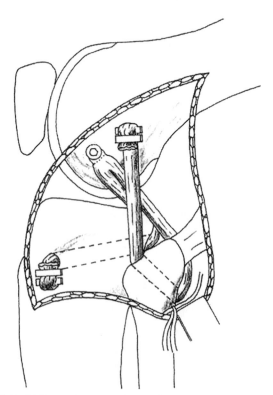

Fig. 7. Reconstruction of LCL, popliteus tendon, and popliteal fibula ligament. (*From* Lee MC, Park YK, Lee SH, et al. Posterolateral reconstruction using split achilles tendon allograft. Arthroscopy 2003;19:1046; with permission.)

popliteal fibular ligament (**Fig. 6**). Lee uses a split Achilles tendon allograft to recon-struct both the PCL, LCL popliteal fibula ligament and popliteus tendon with 1 graft (**Fig. 7**).[23]

When the lateral instability is combined with PCL instability, multiple allografts or au-tografts are needed to reconstruct the PCL and lateral side injury simultaneously. The need for multiple grafts of sufficient size, strength, and length is an excellent reason to choose an allograft for these complex reconstructions. Often times there are insuffi-cient autograft tissues available to accomplish the needed repairs. Allografts also have the advantage of not causing the increased surgical time and morbidity that accompany autograft harvest.

When a lateral side ligament injury is combined with an anterior cruciate tear, the safest approach is to repair the lateral structures with direct suture and soft tissue augmentation, if necessary. After the lateral repair is sufficiently healed and a full range of motion is obtained, the ACL is reconstructed as a second procedure. Staging the surgeries will minimize the risk of arthrofibrosis without compromising the results.

Rehabilitation of both acute and chronic reconstructions of the lateral and postero-lateral corner involves protected weight bearing with early range of motion. Active hamstring use is avoided for at least 12 weeks, because of the stress placed on the posterolateral corner by the biceps pull. Early protected weight bearing can be allowed as soon as muscle tone is adequate to stabilize the knee dynamically, but running should be delayed for approximately 6 months and return to sports for 1 year after these very complex surgical reconstructions.

REFERENCES

1. Woo SL, Inoue M, McGurk-Burleson E, et al. Treatment of the medial collateral ligament injury, II: structure and function of canine knees in response to differing treatment regimens. Am J Sports Med 1987;15:22–9.
2. Indelicato PA. Non-operative treatment of complete tears of the medial collateral ligament of the knee. J Bone Joint Surg Am 1983;65:323–9.
3. Hughston JC, Eilers AF. The role of the posterior oblique ligament in repairs of acute medial (collateral) ligament tears of the knee. J Bone Joint Surg Am 1973;55:923–40.
4. Warren LF, Marshall JL, Girgis F. The prime static stabilizer of the medial side of the knee. J Bone Joint Surg Am 1974;56:665–74.
5. Shelbourne KD, Porter DA. Anterior cruciate ligament-medial collateral ligament injury: non-operative management of medial collateral ligament tears with anterior cruciate ligament reconstruction. Am J Sports Med 1992;20:283–6.
6. Adachi N, Ochi M, Deie M, et al. New hamstring fixation technique for medial col-lateral ligament or posterolateral corner reconstruction using the mosaicplasty system. Arthroscopy 2006;22. 571.e1–3.
7. Horibe S, Shino K, Nagano J, et al. Replacing the medial collateral ligament with an allogenic tendon graft: an experimental canine study. J Bone Joint Surg Br 1990;72B:1044–9.
8. Yoshiya S, Kuroda R, Mizuno K, et al. Medial collateral ligament reconstruction us-ing autogenous hamstring tendons. Technique and results in initial cases. Am J Sports Med 2005;33:1380–5.
9. Hughston JC, Andrews JR. The importance of the posterior oblique ligament in repairs of acute tears of the medial ligament sin knees with and without an asso-ciated rupture of the anterior cruciate ligament. Results of long-term follow-up. J Bone Joint Surg 1994;76(9):1328–44.

10. Wahl CJ, Nicandri G. Single-Achilles allograft posterior cruciate ligament and medial collateral ligament reconstruction: a technique to avoid osseous tunnel intersection, improve construct stiffness, and save on allograft utilization. Arthroscopy 2008;24:486–9.

11. Borden PS, Kantaras AT, Caborn DN. Medial collateral ligament reconstruction with allograft using a double-bundle technique. Arthroscopy 2002;18(4):E19.

12. Coobs BR, LaPrade RF, Griffith CJ, et al. Biomechanical analysis of an isolated fibular (lateral) collateral ligament reconstruction using an autogenous semitendinosus graft. Am J Sports Med 2007;35:1521–7.

13. Latimer HA, Tibone JE, ElAttrache NS, et al. Reconstruction of the lateral collateral ligament of the knee with patellar tendon allograft. Report of a new technique in combined ligament injuries. Am J Sports Med 1998;25:656–62.

14. Noyes FR, Barber-Westin SD. Posterolateral knee reconstruction with an anatomical bone-patellar tendon-bone reconstruction of the fibular collateral ligament. Am J Sports Med 2007;35:259–73.

15. Chen CH, Chen WJ, Shih CH. Lateral collateral ligament reconstruction using quadriceps tendon-patellar bone autograft with bioscrew fixation. Arthroscopy 2001;17(5):551–4.

16. Müller W. The knee: form, function, and ligament reconstruction. Berlin: Springer-Verlag; 1983.

17. Markolf KL, Graves BR, Sigward SM, et al. Popliteus bypass and popliteofibular ligament reconstructions reduce posterior tibial translations and forces in a posterior cruciate ligament graft. Arthroscopy 2007;23:482–7.

18. Nau T, Chevalier Y, Hagemeister N, et al. Comparison of 2 surgical techniques of posterolateral corner reconstruction of the knee. Am Journal Sports Med 2005;33: 1838–45.

19. Larson RV, Sidles JA, Beals TC. Isometry of the lateral collateral and popliteofibular ligaments and a technique for reconstruction. Univ Wash Orthop Res Rep 1996;42–4.

20. Kocabey Y, Nawab A, Caborn DV, et al. Posterolateral corner reconstruction using a hamstring allograft and a bioabsorbable tenodesis screw: description of a new surgical technique. Arthroscopy 2004;20:159–63.

21. Arciero RA. Anatomic posterolateral corner knee reconstruction. Arthroscopy 2005;21:1147. e1–5.

22. Kim SJ, Park IS, Cheon YM, et al. New technique for chronic posterolateral instability of the knee: posterolateral reconstruction using the tibialis posterior tendon allograft. Arthroscopy 2004;20:195–200.

23. Lee MC, Park YK, Lee SH, et al. Posterolateral reconstruction using split Achilles tendon allograft. Arthroscopy 2003;19:1043–9.

Anatomic Double-Bundle Revision Anterior Cruciate Ligament Surgery Using Fresh-Frozen Allograft Tissue

Robert N. Royalty, MD[a], David M. Junkin, Jr., MD[b],
Darren L. Johnson, MD[c],*

KEYWORDS

• Allograft • Revision • Anterior cruciate ligament

Anterior cruciate ligament (ACL) reconstruction is one of the most frequently performed orthopedic procedures. Over the last several decades, the numbers of ACL reconstructions have steadily increased, with estimates of more than 250,000 annually.[1] The American Board of Orthopaedic Surgeons 2003 data from Part-II Certification indicate that primary arthroscopic ACL reconstruction ranks the sixth most common procedure performed overall, even above total knee and hip replacements.[2] Despite increased understanding of knee anatomy and kinematics as well as improved surgical techniques, increasing numbers of primary ACL reconstructions will lead to a concomitant increased incidence in failed primary ACL reconstructions. The incidence of revision surgery for failed primary ACL reconstruction is estimated to be approximately 3% to 25% annually in the United States.[3] The true number of "failures" is unknown. If we look at the number of athletes who return to their sport at the same level of function before their injury, this number may approach 40%. The most common causes of failure are attributed to improper tunnel placement, leading to recurrent instability, persistent postoperative pain, loss of motion, and dysfunction of the extensor mechanism.[4,5] Subjective and objective outcomes of revision ACL reconstruction do not compare with primary reconstruction results, with only approximately 60% of patients returning to the pre-injury level of activity.[4]

[a] Department of Orthopaedic Surgery, University of Kentucky, 740 South Limestone, Suite K401 Kentucky Clinic, Lexington, KY 40536, USA
[b] Department of Orthopaedic Surgery, University of Kentucky, Orthopaedic Specialty Center, Willow Grove, PA 19090, USA
[c] Department of Orthopaedic Surgery, Sports Medicine, University of Kentucky, Lexington, KY 40536, USA
* Corresponding author. Department of Orthopaedic Surgery, University of Kentucky, 740 South Limestone, Suite K401 Kentucky Clinic, Lexington, KY 40536.
E-mail address: dljohns@uky.edu (D.L. Johnson).

Clin Sports Med 28 (2009) 311–326
doi:10.1016/j.csm.2008.10.006
0278-5919/08/$ – see front matter © 2009 Elsevier Inc. All rights reserved.

Once "failure" of primary ACL reconstruction has been established and revision surgery deemed necessary, numerous graft options are available. Similar to primary ACL reconstruction surgery, the choice of graft(s) for revision ACL procedure may include autograft(s) and/or allograft(s). The literature does not clearly support the superiority of one graft option over another, so selection of graft depends on a variety of patient and surgeon variables. Patient preference and surgeon experience/training undoubtedly influence the ultimate decision regarding revision graft selection. Specific variables affecting graft selection that are based on primary ACL reconstruction include source of prior graft, fixation technique, and presence of bone deficiency. Bone-to-bone incorporation of graft material is currently accepted as the biological gold standard for primary and revision ACL reconstruction surgery. Many high-volume primary ACL reconstruction surgeons (including the senior author, DLJ) attempt to avoid the use of all soft-tissue grafts in the young, athletically active patient because of the overall decreased size and lack of bone-to-bone incorporation. The use of fresh-frozen allograft tissue remains the number one graft of choice for revision ACL reconstruction. This article defines the approach to the failed ACL-deficient knee with anterolateral rotatory laxity using allograft tissue as a graft substitute.

Revision ACL reconstruction presents many technical considerations not seen in primary ACL reconstruction. Surgical considerations include, but are not limited to, the location of previous skin incisions, retained hardware, tunnel expansion and bone loss, poor bone quality, prior graft selection, graft fixation issues, concomitant pathology (ie, secondary restraints), and altered postoperative rehabilitation.[6] The extent of tunnel expansion and the position of the previous tunnels significantly influence the selected surgical approach. The question of bone grafting in a single stage versus a two-stage procedure is largely unanswered. The etiology of failure for the primary ACL reconstruction and pre-operative planning are crucial to avoid surgical pitfalls. The etiology of failure for the primary ACL reconstruction and meticulous preoperative planning are crucial to maximize outcome.

Oftentimes, the cause of failure of primary reconstruction remains unclear and is likely multi-factorial. A meticulous pre-operative evaluation, including history, physical examination, and radiographic evaluation, is essential for a successful outcome. Standing anteroposterior (AP) and lateral, weight-bearing 45° flexion posteroanterior (PA), and axial views of the knee assess extremity alignment, notch geometry, coexistent pathology (ie, degenerative joint disease, patella alignment and positions), size and position of tunnels, and fixation technique/implant(s) used in the primary ACL reconstruction (**Fig. 1**). A three-dimensional computed tomography (3D CT) scan of the knee may be necessary to accurately define previous tunnel location, the extent of tunnel expansion, and presence of cystic changes, which may require staging the revision procedure with an initial debridement and bone grafting (**Fig. 2**). Magnetic resonance imaging (MRI) is commonly used to evaluate not only the integrity of the graft but also the other supporting structures and to identify associated pathology (ie, collateral ligaments, menisci, and articular cartilage) that may need to be addressed at the time of revision surgery.

In addition to surgical details, importance of the patient–physician relationship in revision ACL reconstruction cannot be underestimated. Communication between patient and surgeon is vital, especially with regard to expectations. The patient must understand that the goals of revision ACL surgery may often be quite different from primary ACL reconstruction. The goals of primary ACL reconstruction are to prevent further knee injury and allow return to previous levels of activity. Following primary ACL reconstruction, sufficient graft incorporation and return of muscular strength and endurance can largely be achieved by 6 months postoperatively, allowing an athlete to

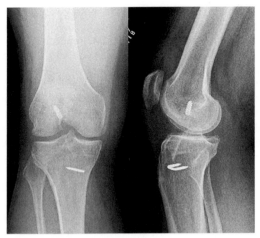

Fig. 1. Preoperative weight-bearing radiographs showing a nonanatomic vertical/anterior-placed femoral graft with a tibial tunnel in the most anterior aspect of the tibial ACL footprint.

return to play "ACL-dependent" sports. For most patients undergoing revision for failed primary ACL surgery, the goal is to eliminate instability interfering with activities of daily living.

The patient's current lifestyle and future plans affect surgical decisions. Surgeons must provide patients with treatment options and allow participation in treatment decisions. Pre-operative education regarding expected time commitment and strict adherence to rehabilitation protocols (ie, brace wear, weight-bearing status, and return to ACL-dependent activities) establishes the importance of the patient's role in overall outcome. The patient and family must understand that healing and graft incorporation in revision surgery may be prolonged compared with primary ACL reconstruction. As such, the patient should not expect to return to ACL-dependent activities until 9 to 12 months after revision ACL reconstruction.

ALLOGRAFT TISSUES

A variety of allograft options are available for use during revision ACL reconstruction including bone-patella tendon-bone, calcaneus-Achilles tendon, and all soft-tissue

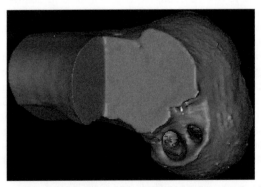

Fig. 2. 3D CT scan showing anatomic double bundle tunnels on the lateral wall of the intercondylar notch.

grafts (quadruple hamstring, quadriceps tendon, anterior tibial tendon, posterior tibial tendon). The 2 most commonly used allografts for revision ACL reconstruction are bone-patella tendon-bone and calcaneus-Achilles tendon. These grafts have peer-reviewed literature to support their use, whereas all soft-tissue allografts currently have minimal support.

Fresh-frozen allograft used for revision ACL reconstruction has several advantages and peer-reviewed literature support. Although allograft tissue is costly, Cole and colleagues[7] found that when comparing bone-patella tendon-bone autograft versus freeze-dried Achilles tendon-bone allograft in primary ACL reconstruction, allograft tissues demonstrate decreased hospital costs through shorter operative, anesthetic, and recovery room times. Ahn and colleagues[8] compared clinical (Lysholm score, International Knee Documentation Committee [IKDC] and stability [KT-2000 arthrometer]) outcome measures of revision ACL reconstruction between different graft materials (quadruple hamstring autograft, bone-patella tendon-bone allograft, Achilles tendon-bone allograft) and did not find any significant difference between graft materials. Fromm and colleagues[9] in a rabbit model established that cryopreserved allografts re-innervate with all 3 types of nerve fibers found in the native ACL by the 24th postoperative week. Shino and colleagues[10] demonstrated that allograft tissue at 6 months showed a blood flow level equivalent to normal control ACLs and histologically reached stability at 18 months post-implantation. Noyes and Barber-Westin[11] studied outcomes of bone-patellar tendon-bone allografts and autografts used for revision ACL reconstruction and found improvements in all patient symptoms, functional limitations, AP displacements, pivot-shift tests, and overall rating scores. Donor-site morbidity from graft harvest, including patella tendon rupture, patella fracture, and anterior knee pain after bone-patella tendon-bone autograft, or hamstring pain and decreased knee flexion strength after hamstring autograft are nonexistent with allografts. Consequently, manual laborers, athletes, or religious sects requiring prolonged kneeling or deep knee bending may benefit from allograft tissue.[12] Autograft tissue is finite; therefore, multi-ligament knee reconstructions requiring significant amounts of tissue for grafts may be ideal for allograft. Additionally, there is no size limitation with allografts; as a result, virtually any tissue-size specification can be met. Lack of size limitation may be the most important variable of why allograft tissue is the graft of choice in revision ACL surgery. With regard to revision ACL reconstruction where hamstring or bone-patella tendon-bone autografts have been previously harvested, allografts are beneficial in preventing additional sacrifice of native tissue. Allograft tissue use significantly decreases operative time with associated smaller incisions and diminish trauma to host tissues, leading to improved cosmesis and decreased pain. In summary, allograft tissues provide significant flexibility for the surgeon involved in revision ACL reconstruction where many unexpected intra-operative challenges must be anticipated.

There are several disadvantages to consider when using allograft tissue in ACL reconstruction. Allograft tissues have the potential for disease transmission as well as immunologic response by host cells, making immunocompromised patients less than ideal candidates for ACL reconstruction via allograft tissues. Grossman and colleagues[13] found greater laxity (increased KT-1000 side-to-side displacement) in knees using allograft tissue (bone-patella tendon-bone and Achilles) versus contralateral bone-patella tendon-bone autograft in revision ACL reconstruction. Shino and colleagues[14] established that fresh-frozen ACL allografts (Achilles, tibialis anterior and posterior, peroneus longus, and brevis) have a collagen fibril profile consisting of predominantly small-diameter collagen fibrils and a decreased number of large-diameter collagen fibrils, which do not resemble the native ACL. Malinin and colleagues[15] performed a human ACL allograft retrieval study examining gross and histologic archi-tecture, demonstrating at 2 years after transplantation that the central portions of the allografts remained acellular and that complete attachment was not present. Mura-matsu and colleagues[16] compared bone-patellar tendon-bone autografts and allo-grafts using contrast-enhanced MRI, finding allogeneic tissues to have a slower onset and rate of revascularization.

In summary, allograft tissues offer several advantages that are particularly relevant in revision ACL reconstruction. For the patient, these include lack of donor site mor-bidity, smaller incisions, and decreased operative time. For the surgeon, the increased tissue availability, variable graft sizes, and the ability to create larger bone plugs pro-vides improved flexibility. This flexibility can be highly beneficial when dealing with complex revision cases that often have unexpected intra-operative challenges. Although allograft tissue may be an invaluable resource in revision cases, the combi-nation of extended incorporation and healing times associated with improved post-operative pain and early function may result in the late sequelae of "laxity" in young, active patients who return to level-1 sports in 6 months.

CALCANEUS-ACHILLES TENDON

Calcaneus-Achilles tendon allograft remains the preferred graft of choice in revision ACL reconstruction. Currently, over 400 patients are waiting for fresh-frozen calca-neus-Achilles tendon grafts from the Musculoskeletal Transplant Foundation (MTF). Calcaneus-Achilles tendon allograft tissue provides abundant bone stock and a long, broad tendinous portion, combining the advantages of bone and soft-tissue grafts. The combination of bone and tendinous attachments permits the Achilles ten-don allograft to be reversed, allowing the gold-standard bone-to-bone fixation in the tibial metaphysis, the most common location of failure and considered the "weak link" in ACL reconstruction. The calcaneal bone attachment of the Achilles tendon al-lograft provides more than enough bone to construct or "customize" a bone block of satisfactory shape and size to "fill" the revision tunnel(s), if needed. The calcaneal bone block can also provide particulate graft for underestimated tunnel expansion, which can be used in staging ACL revision surgery. The abundant tendinous portion of the Achilles tendon allograft provides versatility in sizing, leading to optimal length customization, which may especially be required if one needs to place the graft in the "over-the-top" position on the femur because of tunnel blowout.

BONE-PATELLAR TENDON-BONE ALLOGRAFT

Uribe and colleagues[17] compared fresh-frozen patellar tendon allografts and auto-grafts in revision ACL reconstruction, finding functionally no significant difference in stability between the 2 groups. Bone-patellar tendon-bone allograft offers the advan-tage of 2 bone plugs, providing rigid fixation via the biologic gold standard of bone-to-bone healing. Similar to calcaneus-Achilles tendon allograft, the bone ends are of sufficient size to fashion bone blocks of varying shapes and sizes to accommodate the larger tunnel diameters frequently needed in revision ACL reconstruction, specif-ically "customizing" the graft for that particular patient.

ALL SOFT-TISSUE GRAFTS (ANTERIOR/POSTERIOR TIBIALIS TENDONS, QUADRICEPS TENDON)

Rodeo and colleagues[18] found that soft-tissue grafts require increased time to be incorporated into host tissue based on histologic and biomechanical characteristics of the tendon-bone interface. Almqvist and colleagues[19] evaluated the biomechanical properties of the tibialis tendon allograft and found that the maximal load of the single-loop tibialis (anterior and posterior) tendons (1553 ± 62N) was greater than that of bone-patella tendon-bone allografts (1139 ± 99N) and the stiffness was also greater than bone-patella tendon-bone grafts (236 ± 10 N/mm versus 168 ± 13 N/mm). Singhal and colleagues[20] evaluated clinical outcomes (Lysholm knee score, activity level assessment, and IKDC assessment) and failure rates after primary ACL reconstruction via anterior tibialis allograft and discovered a reoperation rate of 38% overall and 55% failure/reoperation rate in patients younger than 25 years. Morphometric and biomechanical studies of the central quadriceps tendon performed by Harris and colleagues[21] demonstrated that tendon failure occurred at 1075 ± 449N, with load-to-tendon failure 1.36 times that of a comparable-width patellar tendon graft. Grafts composed entirely of soft tissue provide a viable option with adequate strength while simultaneously minimizing bone tunnel size often required to avoid erroneously placed primary tunnels in revision ACL reconstruction.

AUTHORS' PREFERENCE OF SURGICAL APPROACH FOR ANTEROLATERAL LAXITY

Graft choice is tailored to the patient and affected by the graft used for the primary reconstruction. If possible, in the high school or collegiate athlete who continues to participate in competitive level-1 sports and has failed a prior allograft reconstruction, the use of autogenous tissue is preferred. In situations involving the recreational athlete, the low-demand patient older than 25 years of age, or the patient who has failed prior autograft use, the use of a Calcaneus-Achilles tendon allograft is preferred for revision surgery. The large size of the Achilles tendon graft is advantageous in revision cases, because the secondary restraints to anterior and anterolateral rotatory translations are often attenuated, which in turn increases the stresses placed on the graft. Both clinical and kinematic studies have demonstrated improved rotational stability with the anatomic double-bundle reconstruction of the ACL compared with the traditional single-bundle endoscopic technique.[22–28] For these reasons, it is the senior author's (DLJ) choice to perform an anatomic double-bundle reconstruction for revision cases.

EXAMINATION UNDER ANESTHESIA

After induction of general anesthesia, a complete examination of the operative and nonoperative knees is performed. Special attention is paid to the degree of anterior and rotatory laxity as demonstrated by the Lachman test and pivot-shift test, respectively. Occasionally, patients present with AP translational stability, but the degree of rotational laxity is severe, with a grade III or IV pivot shift. The importance of examination under anesthesia (EUA) is demonstrated by the presence of isolated rotatory instability, in which the surgeon may perform an augmentation of the primary graft (discussed in the section on augmentation of primary ACL) versus a complete revision. Failure to identify coexistent ligamentous laxity will result in repeat failure of the ACL graft. If additional laxity is identified, the surgeon may choose to stage the reconstruction or address the additional pathologic laxity simultaneously. The longer the length of time between "failure" and revision ACL reconstruction, the more likely the damage to the secondary restraints.

PATIENT SETUP

It is the authors' preference to use a thigh holder on the operative extremity with the end of the bed lowered or removed. The thigh holder is placed as proximal on the thigh as possible with hip flexion at 45° to allow for maximum knee flexion during surgery. Once the leg is positioned in the thigh holder, the surgeon must verify that the knee can be maximally flexed without interference (**Fig. 3**). The nonoperative leg is placed in the lithotomy position in a well-leg holder (sufficiently padded) with the hip maximally externally rotated. The "well" leg must be positioned to not impede any necessary surgical technique (ie, inside-out meniscal repair).

PORTAL PLACEMENT

The primary ACL arthroscopic portals are often not ideal, and new portals should be established. Poor portal placement will increase the difficulty of the case and lead to poor visualization and access to the intra-articular structures. A high and tight lateral portal adjacent to the inferior patella pole and patellar tendon is established and the arthroscope introduced for diagnostic arthroscopy. A complete inventory of the knee must be performed, documenting the condition of cartilage, menisci, primary ACL graft, and indirect signs of secondary restraint laxity, such as the arthroscopic "drive-through," which indicates medial and/or lateral supporting structure incompetence.[31] A central medial portal is established after proper placement is confirmed with the use of an 18-gauge spinal needle placed percutaneously at the joint line. The needle should be directed in an anterior-to-posterior direction intersecting the ACL tibial footprint. The central medial portal is used to debride the infrapatellar fat-pad and intercondylar notch.

After preparation of the intercondylar notch (as discussed below), an accessory medial portal is established. Localization of the accessory medial portal is achieved with an 18-gauge spinal needle placed percutaneously immediately superior to the medial meniscus. The spinal needle tip is advanced to the desired location of the new AM bundle femoral tunnel. The arthroscope, directed medially from the high and tight lateral portal, must confirm that proper placement of the accessory medial portal will allow the passage of a guide pin and reamer for preparation of the femoral tunnels without damaging the medial femoral condyle articular cartilage. The authors prefer to

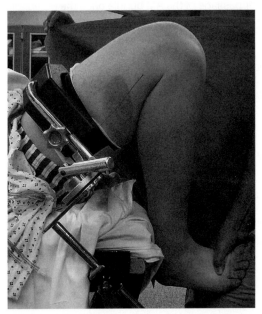

Fig. 3. Patient setup. Note the hyperflexion of knee without interference of the bed. Notice the leg holder is tilted towards the head placing the hip in flexion.

incise the skin in a horizontal fashion for the accessory medial portal, because the instruments introduced through this portal are directed in a medial-to-lateral direction.

GRAFT SELECTION/HARVEST

When performing an anatomic double-bundle reconstruction, the Achilles tendon allograft provides a large soft-tissue graft that may be split into two separate grafts. This technique is cost-effective and eliminates the morbidity of graft harvest (**Fig. 4**). The larger of the two grafts is used for the anteromedial (AM) bundle and the smaller graft to reconstruct the posterolateral (PL) bundle. The bone plug may be retained on the larger AM graft and shaped for tunnel fixation. The excess bone may also be used for bone grafting. If necessary, the Achilles allograft may also be placed in a reverse fashion with the bone plug within the tibial tunnel.[29] In the presence of tibial tunnel expansion, the added volume of bone provides stability and serves to fill tibial metaphyseal defects.

An alternative to splitting the Achilles tendon into two individual grafts is the use of a gracilis tendon autograft for the PL bundle. This technique enables use of the gracilis autograft for the PL bundle and reservation of the entire Achilles allograft for the AM bundle. The use of a hamstring autograft for a revision reconstruction may present difficulties: the gracilis tendon may not be available, having been harvested during primary ACL reconstruction; scar tissue from prior surgery may not allow identification or harvesting of the gracilis tendon without damaging structural integrity; or the pes anserine and its tendinous insertions may have been damaged during primary ACL reconstruction tibial tunnel preparation.

If the gracilis tendon is available, the graft is fashioned in a double-strand technique with an EndoButton (Smith & Nephew, Andover, MA) for femoral fixation. The Achilles graft can be prepared according to the surgeon's preference. It is preferable to remove the Achilles tendon bone plug and prepare the AM bundle as an all soft-tissue graft, allowing easier passage of the AM bundle once the PL bundle has been passed. However, retaining the Achilles tendon bone plug may increase the strength of the

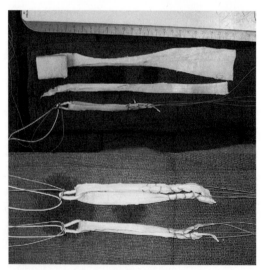

Fig. 4. Calcaneus-Achilles tendon allograft split into two separate grafts for the anteromedial (*top*) and posterolateral (*bottom*) bundles.

femoral fixation, particularly if the newly created AM revision femoral tunnel communicates with the previous primary femoral tunnel. Fortunately, the original femoral tunnels are often placed in a nonanatomic vertical position and can be avoided as the new revision tunnels are placed lower on the lateral femoral wall in the anatomic footprints of the ACL.[30]

INTERCONDYLAR NOTCH PREPARATION

If the primary ACL graft is disrupted or deemed incompetent, the majority of the graft is removed. If a previous screw is present, determination is made whether the hardware may be retained or interferes with revision tunnel placement. If the hardware does not interfere with drilling of the "new" revision femoral tunnels, the hardware is left in place. Retaining hardware eliminates the need for bone grafting any defects and will not weaken the integrity of the lateral femoral condyle. If the hardware must be removed for tunnel preparation, the entire screw head must be exposed with the use of osteotomes and curets to prevent stripping or breakage of the screw. Once the screw is removed, the defect can be filled with excess bone from the calcaneus-Achilles tendon-bone allograft.

Removing as little bone as possible, the notchplasty must provide visualization of the "over-the-top" position within the posterior femoral notch. Likewise, the wallplasty must allow for adequate lateral wall visualization (ie, lateral intercondylar ridge) while minimizing bone removal within the intercondylar notch. It is important to perform a notchplasty only to provide the visualization necessary to anatomically place the femoral tunnels and prevent bony roof impingement on the grafts during knee extension. Removal of more bone than necessary will make proper tunnel placement difficult, because anatomic landmarks may become less identifiable.[32,33] Additionally, removal of excess bone from the lateral wall changes the normal bony attachment site of the ACL, which may adversely affect knee kinematics.

TUNNEL PLACEMENT AND DRILLING

Once the notchplasty and wallplasty are completed, with the knee in 90° of flexion, an awl placed through the accessory medial portal is used to localize the anatomic starting points for both the AM and PL femoral tunnels (**Fig. 5**).[32,33] If the anatomic revision femoral tunnels overlap, which is rare, several options are available. The primary implants can be removed and eccentric tunnel expansion may be considered. If this option is selected, larger bone plugs or adjuvant bone grafting may be required. Another commonly used technique is tunnel divergence: placement of anatomic femoral tunnels via the accessory medial portal results in divergent tunnels that do not communicate with the previously malpositioned primary femoral tunnel, likely originally drilled from a transtibial approach.

The femoral tunnels are prepared via the half-fluted reamer, from the accessory medial portal in standard fashion first, with knee flexion at 110° for the 5- to 6-mm PL tunnel and secondly with knee flexion at 130° for the 7- to 9-mm AM tunnel (**Fig. 6**). This greatly reduces the risk of fracture of the posterior femoral wall and helps in achieving maximal tunnel length. It is preferable to secure the PL bundle with an EndoButton and the AM bundle with an interference screw.

The tibial tunnels are created after preparation of the femoral tunnels. The central medial portal is used for placement of the elbow guide or tibial tip guide to locate proper intra-articular position of the tibial tunnels. Guide pins are passed until the tips are intra-articular. The guide is typically set at 45° and 55° for the PL and AM bundles, respectively. The PL tibial tunnel is placed medial to the AM tunnel at the anterior

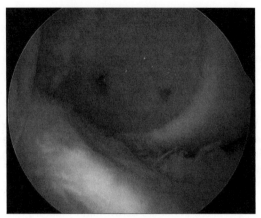

Fig. 5. Anatomic starting point for AM and PL bundles marked with an awl at 90° of flexion as viewed from accessory medial portal.

edge of the medial collateral ligament (MCL) on the proximal tibial metaphysis. The guide pins should be centered in the anatomic footprint of the respective bundle **(Fig. 7)**.[32,33] As is commonly the case on the tibial side, the primary ACL tibial tunnel may need to be used, typically for the AM tunnel. It is recommended to remove all remnants of the prior graft and then expand the tibial tunnel in the appropriate direction to achieve the desired location. Creating the ideal tibial tunnel can be achieved by placing a guide pin by hand through the primary ACL tibial tunnel and securing the tip of the pin in the roof of the femoral notch to maintain the guide pin position. A cannulated drill/reamer or dilator can then be used for directed expansion of the tunnel. The process will need to be repeated until anatomic placement of the tunnel has been achieved. In our experience, communication of the 2 tibial tunnels at the articular surface, which is quite common, will not affect the placement of the grafts or fixation.

GRAFT PASSAGE AND FIXATION

The grafts are passed using a passing pin and sutures in standard fashion. The pin is first passed through the accessory inferomedial portal and up the femoral tunnel with

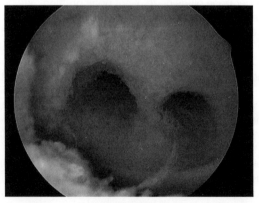

Fig. 6. Anatomic AM and PL tunnels at 90° of flexion as viewed from accessory medial portal.

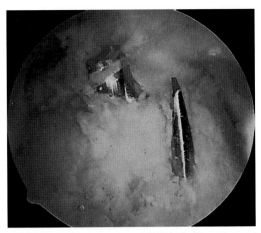

Fig. 7. Tibial entry sites marked by pin (AM) and drill (PL) through previous tunnel opening at the level of the joint line.

the knee flexed to approximately 120°. A suture loop is pulled into the knee with the pin, and hyperflexion is released. The suture loop is grasped with a pituitary passed up through the tibial tunnel and subsequently pulled out of this tunnel. The loop is used to pass graft sutures through both tunnels and out of the anterolateral aspect of the knee. The graft is then advanced into place. For the double-bundle reconstruction, the PL (all soft-tissue) graft is generally passed first and fixed on the femoral side before passing the larger AM graft (**Fig. 8**). In those cases where a single, expanded tibial tunnel has been created we hold the PL bundle in the posterior aspect of the tibial tunnel while passing the AM bundle to ensure appropriate orientation (**Fig. 9**).

In most cases, femoral side fixation is performed using a cannulated bioabsorbable (polylactide carbonate) interference screw(s) (Smith & Nephew, Andover, MA). Once the graft has been secured to the femoral side, the knee is cycled to pretension the graft(s). The knee is then brought into full extension for tibial side fixation. If two separate tibial tunnels were created for the double-bundle reconstruction the bundles are

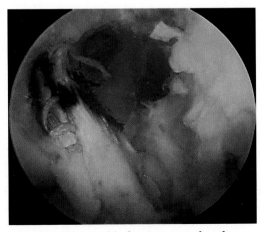

Fig. 8. PL bundle with empty AM tunnel before passage of graft.

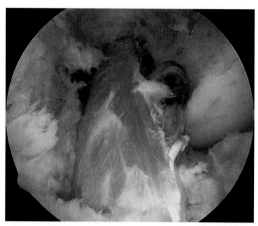

Fig. 9. View from the accessory medial portal with the knee at 90° of flexion after the passage of the grafts.

typically tensioned and fixed with the knee in different positions. The PL bundle is fixed with the knee in full extension, while the AM bundle is set with the knee in approximately 30° to 60° of flexion. Bioabsorbable interference screws and back-up fixation is typically used in most cases. The interference screw is usually sized to match or one size larger than the last tibial tunnel reamer. Back-up fixation is achieved with a staple or screw and spiked washer.

Once graft fixation has been completed, the graft(s) is inspected to ensure there is no impingement from the wall or notch. The arthroscope is then reinserted into the tight medial portal to confirm graft position and orientation from an on-face perspective. Repeat examination of the knee is performed in the operating room with the Lachman, anterior drawer, and pivot-shift tests.

SURGICAL PEARLS AND PITFALLS

The quality of the patient's bone and the location of the bone tunnels from the primary surgery are uncontrollable variables. The use of half-size dilators may be particularly important in the preparation of tibial and femoral tunnels in patients with poor bone quality. In preparation of the bone tunnels in either the tibia or the femur, the use of half-size dilators may become important. With poor bone quality, dilators allow expansion of the tunnel to the desired diameter without removing any additional bone. If simultaneous bone grafting is undertaken, the dilators aid in impacting the bone graft material, particularly if the area being grafted communicates with the newly created revision tunnel. Note, when communication between tunnels occurs, interference screw fixation may not provide secure fixation; therefore, EndoButton or metaphyseal fixation are alternatives.

Tibial fixation ("weak link") remains a concern in the primary reconstruction and even more so in the revision case. The additional length afforded by the allograft will allow for additional fixation at the tibial metaphysis. Interference screw fixation in the PL tibial tunnel may not be an option given the small diameter of the graft and tunnel (averaging 6 to 7 mm); therefore, staple fixation is commonly used. For additional stabilization, a large staple can be placed distally to secure both the AM and PL grafts, after an interference screw has been placed in the AM tibial tunnel. The surgeon must be prepared to use interference screws, staples, screws with a spiked washer, or a combination of fixation devices to ensure stable tibial fixation (**Fig. 10**).

AUGMENTATION OF PRIMARY ACL

Many traditional endoscopic single-bundle reconstructions with "failed" results because of rotatory laxity may have an intact primary ACL graft without demonstration of anterior laxity on EUA and arthroscopic inspection. Retention of the primary ACL graft and augmentation with a second bundle is a treatment alternative. A single bundle placed within the femur in either the 11 or 1 o'clock position can be retained if providing AP stability and augmented with a graft placed in an anatomic position on the femoral wall, to provide rotational stability.[34] Results of such an augmenting procedure are unknown. Augmentation must be approached with caution. The previous graft must be intact, provide stability to the knee in the AP direction, and must have the "normal" arthroscopic appearance on visualization. The augmentation can then be customized to fit the need of the patient, restoring stability by replacement of either AM or PL bundles.

Commonly, the previous graft was placed in a vertical position, originating from the PL insertion on the tibia to the 11 or 1 o'clock position on the femur. This allows for the placement of an "augmenting" graft or bundle in a horizontal or anatomic position. The new tibia tunnel can be positioned anteriorly on the tibial articular surface within the footprint of the AM bundle, and a new femoral tunnel can be placed "lower" on the lateral femoral wall, without disrupting the primary graft. The new anatomic bundle restores rotational stability to the knee.

If the prior graft was placed anteriorly on the tibial articular surface, the surgeon may choose to augment with an anatomically placed PL bundle. This procedure may be difficult to perform because the primary ACL graft blocks visualization of the exit point of the new PL tibial tunnel. After placement of the guide pin via the tibial guide, one

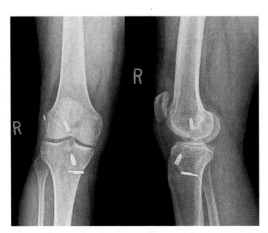

Fig. 10. Weight-bearing radiographs one year after revision anatomic double-bundle revision reconstruction. AM bundle fixation was provided with bioabsorbable interference screws and the PL bundle fixation via an EndoButton (Smith & Nephew, Andover, MA) and staple. The metal interference screw within the femur was retained from the primary surgery, because the primary nonanatomic femoral tunnel did not interfere with the position of the anatomic revision tunnels. The previous tibial tunnel was used for the PL graft, and a new AM tibial tunnel was drilled.

must be sure that drilling a new tunnel will not disrupt the primary graft. If the previous graft will not allow for the desired placement of the new tunnels or disruption of the primary graft occurs, converting to a formal revision reconstruction is recommended as previously described.

REHABILITATION

Postoperative rehabilitation after revision ACL reconstruction should be tailored to the surgical procedure as well as specific patient factors. Important surgical factors to consider include type of graft (allograft versus autograft), type of fixation, concomitant procedures (ie, reconstruction/augmentation of secondary restraints, osteotomy, meniscal repair/transplantation), and associated laxity of secondary restraints. Patient considerations include age, activity level, size, compliance of the patient, and expectations. Rehabilitation protocols for revision ACL reconstruction are less aggressive than primary ACL surgery, especially in patients in whom the revision is considered a "salvage" operation. In such circumstances, the goals of rehabilitation are to restore a stable and functional knee for activities of daily living and occupational demands.

The first week of rehabilitation focuses on decreasing swelling and inflammation. Immediate full weight bearing as tolerated is allowed with the hinged knee brace locked in full extension. Typically, the hinged knee brace is locked in extension during ambulation for 1 month postoperatively. Protecting revision patients in a hinged knee brace while upright and ambulating for approximately 2 months following reconstruction is preferred. A focus on obtaining full range of motion by 4 to 6 weeks postoperatively remains, while the time frame for progression through functional exercises and strengthening is tailored to the patient. Return to sport criteria are similar to primary procedures but often should be delayed for at least 9 to 12 months postoperatively.

SUMMARY

Autograft tissue is finite. There are no size limitations with allografts; as a result, virtually any tissue-size specification can be met, tailoring the graft to the needs and demands of the patient. Allografts are also beneficial in preventing additional sacrifice of native tissue. Autogenous tissues may be limited secondary to multiple factors, including their use during the primary reconstruction, scar formation, or size and amount of tissue that can be feasibly harvested. Allograft tissue use significantly decreases operative time with associated smaller incisions and diminishes trauma to host tissues, leading to improved cosmesis and decreased pain. Unlike autografts, allograft tissue dimensions may be specified to provide additional length and diameter of the tissue for better fill within the bony tunnels. The added length may be beneficial with regard to fixation at the femoral and tibial sides. The Achilles tendon-bone and bone-patellar tendon-bone allografts provide a large bony plug not only for bone grafting pre-existing osseous defects but also allow one to shape the osseous plug to provide adequate fill in a previous bone tunnel that may have expanded via osteolysis. The appropriate use of allograft tissues provides significant flexibility for the surgeon involved in revision of failed primary ACL reconstruction using an anatomic double-bundle technique.

REFERENCES

1. Marrale J, Morrissey MC, Haddad FS, et al. A literature review of autograft and allograft anterior cruciate ligament reconstruction. Knee Surg Sports Traumatol Arthrosc 2007;15(6):690–704. Epub 2007 Apr 12.

2. Garrett WE Jr, Swiontkowski MF, Weinstein JN, et al. American board of orthopaedic surgery practice of the orthopaedic surgeon: part-II, certification examination case mix. J Bone Joint Surg Am 2006;88(3):660–7.
3. Diamantopoulos AP, Lorbach O, Paessler HH, et al. Anterior cruciate ligament revision reconstruction: results in 107 Patients. Am J Sports Med 2008;36:851–60.
4. Battaglia MJ, Cordasco FA, Hannafin JA, et al. Results of revision anterior cruciate ligament surgery. Am J Sports Med 2007;35:2057–66.
5. Harilainen A, Sandelin J. Revision anterior cruciate ligament surgery. A review of the literature and results of our own revisions. Scand J Med Sci Sports 2001;11: 163–9.
6. Safran MR, Harner CD. Technical considerations of revision anterior cruciate ligament surgery. Clin Orthop Relat Res 1996;325:50–64.
7. Cole DW, Ginn TA, Chen GJ, et al. Cost comparison of anterior cruciate ligament reconstruction: autograft versus allograft. Arthroscopy 2005;21(7):786–90.
8. Ahn JH, Lee YS, Ha HC. Comparison of revision surgery with primary anterior cruciate ligament reconstruction and outcome of revision surgery between different graft materials. Amer J Sports Med 2008;1889–96.
9. Fromm B, Schäfer B, Parsch D, et al. Reconstruction of the anterior cruciate ligament with a cryopreserved ACL allograft. A microangiographic and immunohistochemical study in rabbits. Int Orthop 1996;20(6):378–82.
10. Shino K, Inoue M, Horibe S, et al. Surface blood flow and histology of human anterior cruciate ligament allografts. Arthroscopy 1991;7(2):171–6.
11. Noyes FR, Barber-Westin SD. Revision anterior cruciate ligament surgery: experience from Cincinnati. Clin Orthop Relat Res 1996;325:116–29.
12. Strickland SM, MacGillivray JD, Warren RF, et al. Anterior cruciate ligament reconstruction with allograft tendons. Orthop Clin North Am 2003;34(1):41–7.
13. Grossman MG, ElAttrache NS, Shields CL, et al. Revision anterior cruciate ligament reconstruction: three- to nine-year follow-up. Arthroscopy 2005;21(4): 418–23.
14. Shino K, Oakes BW, Horibe S, et al. Collagen fibril populations in human anterior cruciate ligament allografts. Electron microscopic analysis. Am J Sports Med 1995;23(2):203–8 [discussion: 209].
15. Malinin TI, Levitt RL, Bashore C, et al. A study of retrieved allografts used to replace anterior cruciate ligaments. Arthroscopy 2002;18(2):163–70.
16. Muramatsu K, Hachiya Y, Izawa H, et al. Serial evaluation of human anterior cruciate ligament grafts by contrast-enhanced magnetic resonance imaging: comparison of allografts and autografts. Arthroscopy 2008;24(9):1038–44.
17. Uribe JW, Hechtman KS, Zvijac JE, et al. Revision anterior cruciate ligament surgery: experience from Miami. Clin Orthop Relat Res 1996;325:91–9.
18. Rodeo SA, Arnoczky SP, Torzilli PA, et al. Tendon-healing in a bone tunnel. A biomechanical and histological study in the dog. J Bone Joint Surg Am 1993;75(12): 1795–803.
19. Almqvist KF, Jan H, Vercruysse C, et al. The tibialis tendon as a valuable anterior cruciate ligament allograft substitute: biomechanical properties. Knee Surg Sports Traumatol Arthrosc 2007;15(11):1326–30. Epub 2007 Aug 22.
20. Singhal MC, Gardiner JR, Johnson DL, et al. Failure of primary anterior cruciate ligament surgery using anterior tibialis allograft. Arthroscopy 2007;23(5): 469–75.
21. Harris NL, Smith DA, Lamoreaux L, et al. Central quadriceps tendon for anterior cruciate ligament reconstruction. part I: morphometric and biomechanical evaluation. Am J Sports Med 1997;25(1):23–8.

22. Cha PS, Brucker PU, West RV, et al. Arthroscopic double-bundle anterior cruciate ligament reconstruction: an anatomic approach. Arthroscopy 2005;21(10):1275.
23. Buoncristiani AM, Tjoumakaris FP, Starman JS, et al. Anatomic double-bundle anterior cruciate ligament reconstruction. Arthroscopy 2006;22:1000–6.
24. Cohen SB, Starman JB, Fu FH, et al. Anatomical double-bundle anterior cruciate ligament reconstruction. Techniques in Knee Surgery 2006;5:99–106.
25. Muneta T, Koga H, Mochizuki T, et al. A prospective randomized study of 4-strand semitendinosus tendon anterior cruciate ligament reconstruction comparing single-bundle and double-bundle techniques. Arthroscopy 2007;23:618–28.
26. Siebold R, Dehler C, Ellert T, et al. Prospective randomized comparison of double-bundle versus single-bundle anterior cruciate ligament reconstruction. Arthroscopy 2008;24:137–45.
27. Stretch NA, Friedrich K, Gotterbarm T, et al. Reconstruction of the ACL with a semitendinosus tendon graft: a prospective randomized single blinded comparison of double-bundle versus single-bundle technique in male athletes. Knee Surg Sports Traumatol Arthrosc 2008;16(3):232–8. Epub 2008 Jan 12.
28. Yagi M, Kuroda R, Nagamune K, et al. Double-bundle ACL reconstruction can improve rotational stability. Orthop Relat Res 2007;454:100–7.
29. Zamorano DP, Gold SM. Reverse Achilles tendon allograft technique for anterior cruciate ligament reconstruction. Arthroscopy 2005;21:769.e1–3.
30. Stevenson WW, Johnson DL. "Vertical grafts": a common reason for functional failure after ACL reconstruction. Orthopedics 2007;30:206–9.
31. LaPrade RF. Arthroscopic evaluation of the lateral compartment of knees with grade 3 posterolateral knee complex injuries. Am J Sports Med 1997;25(5):596–602.
32. Edwards A, Bull AMJ, Amis AA, et al. The attachments of the anteromedial and posterolateral fiber bundles of the anterior cruciate ligament part 2: femoral attachment. Knee Surg Sports Traumatol Arthrosc 2008;16:29–36.
33. Edwards A, Bull AMJ, Amis AA. The attachments of the anteromedial and posterolateral fiber bundles of the anterior cruciate ligament part 1: tibial attachment. Knee Surg Sports Traumatol Arthrosc 2007;15:1414–21.
34. Brophy RH, Selby RM, Altchek DW, et al. Anterior cruciate ligament revision: double-bundle augmentation of primary vertical graft. Arthroscopy 2006;22:683.e1–5.

Future of Allografts in Sports Medicine

Christopher D. Harner, MD[a,*], Marvin Y. Lo, MD[a,b]

KEYWORDS

• Allograft • Knee • Sports medicine • ACL

In sports medicine, allograft tissues are used for many common and some uncommon procedures. They have become popular choices for surgery, because there are a variety of advantages including increased versatility of the graft, decreased operative time, elimination of harvesting autograft tissue, elimination of autograft morbidity, ease of postoperative recovery, and versatility in complex procedures requiring multiple grafts (as this precludes autograft harvest). They have increasingly been used in ligament reconstruction surgery (anterior cruciate ligament [ACL], posterior cruciate ligament [PCL], and multiligamentous reconstruction), in meniscus transplantation, in osteochondral transplantation, and in the patellofemoral joint with medial patellofemoral ligament (MPFL) reconstruction. The use of musculoskeletal allograft tissue has risen dramatically in the past couple of decades from approximately 350,000 in 1990 to more than 850,000 in 2001.[1] The Musculoskeletal Transplant Foundation (MTF), a not-for-profit organization founded by academic orthopedic surgeons in 1987 and one of many allograft distribution businesses, reported in 2002 that they had procured from 4,431 donors and distributed almost 300,000 units of tissue.[2]

A survey of the American Orthopaedic Society for Sports Medicine (AOSSM) in 2006 regarding allograft usage and concerns indicated that of the 365 respondents, the vast majority (86%) use allografts. However, the vast majority (73%) also reported concerns about the safety of nonsterilized allografts with regard to disease transmission, but most of these respondents (82%) were confident in the safety of sterilized grafts. Additionally, 81% of the respondents reported that they harbored some belief that the tissue quality was compromised to some extent by the sterilization processes. In terms of quality control, 75% of the respondents stated that they use allografts only from tissue banks accredited by the American Association of Tissue Banks (AATB), an organization that sets stringent standards but that is also completely voluntary. Another 21% did not know whether their tissue banks were AATB accredited or not.

[a] UPMC Sports Performance Complex, UPMC Center for Sports Medicine, Department of Orthopaedic Surgery, University of Pittsburgh Medical Center, 3200 S. Water Street, Pittsburgh, PA 15203, USA
[b] Orthopaedic Group of San Francisco, 1700 California St. #300, San Francisco, CA 94109, USA
* Corresponding author.
E-mail address: harnercd@msx.upmc.edu (C.D. Harner).

Clin Sports Med 28 (2009) 327–340
doi:10.1016/j.csm.2008.10.010
0278-5919/08/$ – see front matter © 2009 Elsevier Inc. All rights reserved.

About 46% of these same respondents did not know whether the tissues were sterilized or knew very little about the process itself.[3]

It is clear based on the AOSSM survey that the use of allograft tissue is widespread within the sports community and certainly has increased from a decade ago, although the knowledge of the tissue procurement and sterilization processes and confidence in the mechanical integrity of the soft tissue allografts after irradiation and sterilization are somewhat in question. The widespread usage of allografts in the future of sports medicine is in large part dependent on the ability to gain this knowledge and confidence in the soft tissue procurement and sterilization process. There are many proprietary sterilization procedures in the industry, and many articles have looked at the end sterilization process with gamma irradiation. At issue is the fact that the mechanical integrity of the soft tissue is affected at irradiation levels needed to kill a virus. Therefore, there is a fine balance between maintaining the mechanical properties of the allograft and achieving adequate sterilization of the tissue, and the future role of allografts in sports medicine will depend on the industry's ability to allay the public concern about infection while addressing surgeons' concern about mechanical properties of the implanted grafts. The authors believe that allograft will remain the tissue of choice for meniscus transplant and osteochondral allograft barring the advent of stem cell and genetically engineered implants. Regarding ligament surgery, the authors believe that allograft may remain the ligament of choice for low-energy-type reconstructions such as MPFL reconstructions and in cases where the flexibility and number of grafts preclude autograft harvest (ie, multiligamentous reconstruction). With regard to ACL surgery, the authors prefer autograft for young high-level athletes, because the goal is to get them back in play as early as possible, and the authors have experienced minimal morbidity with autograft harvest and postoperative pain. Recent data from the Multicenter Orthopaedic Outcomes Network (MOON) trial presented at the AOSSM 2008 have raised concerns as to the success of allograft ACL surgery in young patients between ages 10 and 19, and it will be interesting to continue to follow these outcomes.[4]

ALLOGRAFTS

Allograft procurement and use in orthopedic surgery first started in the early 1900s as bone augmentation in spinal fusions and fracture nonunions. The tissue was originally obtained from amputated limbs. During the Korean conflict in the 1950s, the Navy Tissue Bank was formed to satisfy the increasing demand for allograft tissue.[5] The "modern" era of tissue banks started in the 1970s and has evolved with the increase in both organ donors and allograft use in surgery.[6] The original indications for allograft were reserved for complex procedures in which massive grafting was required and autograft was not an option. This has become increasingly popular with studies showing comparable results in soft tissue surgery between allograft and autograft[7,8] along with concerns of donor-site morbidity.[9] Donors have increased in the United States from 6000 in 1996 to more than 22,000 in 2005.[10] Each year approximately 1.5 million bone and soft tissue allografts are implanted, 10% of which are soft tissue grafts.[11] Of the soft tissue grafts implanted, the most commonly used are bone-patellar tendon-bone (BPTB), Achilles tendon, fascia lata, tibialis, quadriceps, hamstring tendons, and meniscus.[12] With the increase in allograft implantation, the importance of regulation in allograft procurement and sterilization cannot be overstated.

Oversight of the tissue banking industry occurs on 3 levels: (1) AATB, (2) Food and Drug Administration (FDA), (3) State-level regulation. Tissue banks oversee donor screening, recovery of body parts, processing, sterilization, storage, and distribution.

In 2001, there were 154 tissue banks, only 36 of which were actually inspected by any of these regulatory agencies, and that has since changed.[13] Efforts to regulate the process have dramatically improved. The FDA implemented requirements for current good tissue practices (CGTP) in May 2005. All tissue banks are required to file with the FDA; the FDA retains the right to inspect all facilities without notice; and the FDA has the ability to issue tissue recalls and even shut down facilities if they do not meet requirements.[14] Additionally, the AATB has come out with its own "Standards for Tissue Banking," now on the 11th edition published in 2006.[15] Although the organization is voluntary, the American Academy of Orthopaedic Surgeons (AAOS) has stated in multiple position papers to its members that "all tissue banks should follow national guidelines and standards, and allografts should only come from AATB accredited tissue banks." According to the AOSSM survey, a vast majority of orthopedic surgeons adhere to this.[5] On the state level, only New York and Florida license and inspect tissue banks. California provides licensing but does not inspect tissue banks, and Georgia and Maryland require only registration of tissue banks.[5]

Although tissue procurement and sterilization are continually improving, multiple high-profile cases related to allograft safety have been the focus of public scrutiny in the last decade. Most of these incidents have occurred through either illegal activity or violation of FDA or AATB regulations.

In 2001, a young man in Minnesota underwent surgery for osteochondral allograft implantation, and subsequently developed an allograft-associated infection with *Clostridium sordellii*, which resulted in his death. A second individual was later identified who had also received allograft tissue from the same donor and developed a similar infection, but he was treated successfully with antibiotics. Investigation into this incident revealed that the donor's body was not refrigerated until 19 hours postmortem, and harvesting of the tissues occurred at 24 hours in violation of standard good tissue practice regulations. At the time of occurrence, both the tissue recovery and processing organizations were not part of the AATB, which requires harvest within 15 hours postmortem in nonrefrigerated or cooled cases.[16,17] CryoLife Inc (Kennesaw, GA) was discovered to be the processing and distribution organization, and subsequent investigations revealed 14 other donors who had met the same case procedures. CryoLife was ultimately ordered to recall 7,913 tissue products. They were eventually forced to change their policies and were not cleared to process orthopedic tissues again until 2003.[18]

In 2005 the company Biomedical Tissue Services (BTS), now defunct, likely forged death certificates and tissue donor consent forms and allegedly falsified key information such as serology testing, age, and cause of death. The FDA ordered BTS to cease all activity, and this incident resulted in the recall of approximately 26,000 allografts by 5 tissue banks.[19,20]

In 2006 Donor Referral Services came under scrutiny in newspaper headlines for allegedly falsifying records of donors. It was later reported that the owner had allegedly fabricated donor age, cause of death, and risk factors for communicable diseases in at least 5 donor cases, resulting in notification of hundreds of donors for potential infection.[21]

That same year, 2006, there was yet another incident in the mass media, reported by the Associated Press. This time a woman received an allograft and subsequently developed *Chryseobacterium meningosepticum* infection. She was treated successfully with antibiotics and was able to retain the graft. Tests at the Centers for Disease Control and Prevention (CDC) on the same tissue nonimplanted showed identical bacteria and, therefore, a link was made. The MTF subsequently issued a voluntary recall of 4,700 tissues.[22]

These episodes illustrate the complexity of allograft procurement and sterilization and the difficulty in maintaining good quality control with so many variables, even with the increasingly stringent regulations set forth by the FDA and AATB today.

TISSUE PROCESSING

An understanding of each step in tissue processing is vital to understanding the role that allograft soft tissue now plays and its role in the future of sports medicine. Tissue procurement is the first stage and occurs through recovery from organ donors. Tissues can come from hospital operating rooms or morgues, coroners, or modernized funeral homes, but the vast majority (89%) of tissues are obtained through organ procurement organizations (OPOs).[23] There are around 44 OPOs in the United States, some of which have become tissue banks as well.[24]

The suitability of each donor is determined by a licensed physician. A standard questionnaire assesses risk followed by physical assessment, medical record review, and autopsy review (if performed). Soft tissue donation is automatically rejected if there is a history of autoimmune disease, ingestion of or exposure to toxic substances, rheumatoid arthritis, systemic lupus, polyarteritis nodosa, sarcoidosis, and clinically significant bone disease. Blood is then screened for infectious disease. Donors must test negative for antibodies to human immunodeficiency virus (HIV), and nucleic acid testing (NAT) must be done for HIV-1. Other tests include hepatitis B surface antigen, total antibody to hepatitis B core antigen, antibodies to hepatitis C virus (HCV), NAT for HCV, antibodies to human T-lymphotropic virus, and syphilis. NAT testing is a provision of the AATB as of March 2005 and markedly decreases the window of time for the detection of the viruses.[25]

From the point of infection, there is a window of time during which it is too soon for tests to detect the viruses or antibodies. With NAT, the window period has decreased to approximately 7 days for HIV and HCV and 8 days for hepatitis B virus (HBV).[26] The current risk of transplanting tissue from an HIV-infected donor has been estimated to be between 1 in 173,000 and 1 in 1.1 million.[2,27,28] Overall, the percentage of total donors from which tissue is eventually procured averages 57% but varies significantly by location (9%–92%).[23] Assuming the donor has passed preliminary testing, the tissue excision must then commence within 15 hours of death if the body is nonrefrigerated or within 24 hours if refrigerated.[16] A surgical team harvests the tissue in the standard surgical manner with appropriate prep and drape procedures. The tissue is rapidly cooled to maintain tissue integrity and sterility until further processing can occur. Tissues are normally kept in quarantine up to 5 weeks pending the outcome of all serologic testing.[23]

INFECTION

Infection remains the major concern for allografts, with the 2 most devastating types being HIV and HCV. The risk of HIV transmission is estimated as 1 in 1.6 million.[29] There have been documented cases of HIV resulting from allograft implantation in orthopedic surgery, but none has occurred after implementation of stringent HIV screening practices with polymerase chain reaction (PCR) and NAT.[30] The first incident occurred in 1984 before screening of donors for HIV began. In this case, a young woman received femoral head allograft from an infected donor. This bone was used for spinal fusion in idiopathic scoliosis. The donor had a history of intravenous drug abuse, underwent biopsy for lymphadenopathy before death, and was not screened for HIV. The recipient died from complications related to acquired immunodeficiency syndrome (AIDS).[31] HIV screening started in 1985. In 1992, a second case was reported in a transplantation of bone allograft. The donor was a 22-year-old man with no risk factors and negative serum tests for HIV. In this case, 4 other recipients who received kidneys, liver, and heart from this same donor ultimately became infected. Additionally, 3 recipients of frozen unprocessed musculoskeletal allografts became infected. Another 25 recipients of freeze-dried bone chips, segments of fascia lata, tendon, and ligaments were infected.[30,32]

The risk of hepatitis infection with musculoskeletal allograft is higher than that with HIV: 1 in 421,000.[28] This is likely due to the higher prevalence of hepatitis in this country—up to 3.9 million estimated with hepatitis C alone.[26] While HIV stays in cadaveric blood for up to 48 hours, making it stable for PCR or NAT testing, the hepatitis virus continues to clear from serum after death via the immune system and therefore can have a serum half-life of only a few hours. Therefore, a false negative is possible.[25,33] In Portland, Oregon for example, a donor infected with HCV was not detected, and subsequently, his tissues infected at least 6 patients. On initial donor screening, he was anti-HCV antibody–negative and HCV RNA–positive. Policies have since changed to include PCR and NAT in response.[34]

Bacterial infection is more common than infection with HIV or hepatitis. Although the reporting is completely voluntary, there have been multiple reports in the literature about this. In 2000, 4 case reports detailed septic arthritis following ACL surgery with allograft, and this prompted more stringent sterilization methods. A 16-year-old girl in Florida had bone-tendon-bone (BPTB) allograft with subsequent septic arthritis with *Pseudomonas aeruginosa*, *Staphylococcus aureus*, and *Enterococcus faecalis*–positive cultures. That same month, a 40-year-old man developed septic arthritis in the knee after BPTB allograft ACL with *Pseudomonas aeruginosa* infection. Later on that year (October), a 55-year-old woman with BPTB allograft developed a *Citrobacter werkmanii* and Group B streptococcus septic knee, and again in that same month, a 29-year-old woman also with BPTB allograft developed septic arthritis from *Klebsiella oxytoca* and *Hafnia alvei* infection. Up to March 2003, 26 cases of bacterial infection had been reported in the voluntary reporting system, and 1 patient in Minnesota had died. It should be noted that the bulk of these infections occurred before the usage of terminal sterilization.[5] In response to these episodes, in February 2002 the AAOS formed a Tissue Banking Project Team to work with both the FDA and CDC to help address the issue of allograft safety.

Closer observation of the episodes of infection mentioned here shows that most infections with HIV or hepatitis C occurred toward the beginning of each specific epidemic—in other words, before we adequately understood the pathogen or had adequate testing for it. The implication of this, of course, is that we cannot screen for what we do not know about, and we do not know what the next "hep C" will be. A workshop (titled Blood, Organ, and Other Tissues Safety workshop) was convened in 2005 through the FDA, CDC, and HRSA (Health Resources and Services Administration) to address these issues of allograft safety and the rapid recognition and communication of potential pathogens. This was in response to concerns expressed in the health care industry regarding transmission of pathogens such as Chagas disease, West Nile virus, rabies, and so on. Therefore, it is clear that both the government and orthopedic organizations take the issue of allograft safety very seriously.

STERILIZATION

There is no such thing as a completely sterile tissue. In the organ procurement world, sterility is a mathematical probability. This is measured as SAL (sterility assurance level), and for a tissue to be labeled sterile the SAL must be 10^{-6}, meaning a less than 1 in 1,000,000 chance of a contaminating organism surviving the treatment.[12]

The goal of secondary sterilization is to eliminate all risk of infection while maintaining the biologic and mechanical properties of the graft. There is no perfect method of secondary sterilization today. Earlier methods included ethylene oxide, which was discontinued following a high incidence of mechanical graft failure and chronic synovitis.[35]

Another common method for sterilization is gamma irradiation. This works in 2 ways: (1) generation of free radicals, and (2) direct modification of nucleic acids leading to genomic dysfunction. Bacteria are effectively killed at doses of 1.5 to 2.5 Mrad,[36] but doses higher than 3.5 Mrad are required to kill viruses.[37] The current recommended dose is 2.5 Mrad, because anything above this has been shown to affect the mechanical integrity of the graft.[25]

Gamma irradiation has therefore been combined with other proprietary methods of cleansing, with the actual irradiation reserved for "end irradiation."

As seen here, the required dosage to sterilize the tissue against viruses is too high to maintain the biomechanical integrity of the graft tissue. Thus, there is no ideal sterilization procedure, but multiple different processes are used.

For example, CryoLife Inc (Kennesaw, GA) uses a slow freezing rate with dimethyl sulfoxide (DMSO) or glycerol to cryopreserve the grafts. After swab culturing and desiccation, the grafts are treated in an antimicrobial solution for an extended period of time. BioCleanse (Regeneration Technologies Inc, Alachua, FL) uses low-temperature chemical sterilization, and Allowash (Lifenet, Virginia Beach, VA) uses ultrasonics, centrifugation, and negative pressure in combination with reagents, such as detergents, alcohols, and hydrogen peroxide, to solubilize and remove lipids, marrow cells, and so forth.

Packaging options, much like sterilization options, are varied. They include fresh allograft, fresh freezing, cryopreservation, and lyophilization. Fresh grafts must be implanted shortly after harvest, whereas fresh-frozen grafts can be stored for up to 3 to 5 years in temperatures between -80 to $-196°C$. In cryopreservation, the tissue undergoes controlled-rate freezing with water extraction by glycerol and DMSO. The shelf life approaches 10 years with good cell viability. Freeze-drying or lyophilization is a method whereby the residual moisture is <5%, and the graft can be stored at room temperature.[25]

As seen here, although there are many advantages to the use of allografts, the tissue procurement process itself, along with the sterilization process, is full of variables, which make quality control difficult to oversee. Additionally, while there is a substantial amount of oversight throughout the process, the reports in the lay media and the case reports over the past few years clearly show that human error can significantly change the quality of the tissue endpoint. The future of allografts in sports medicine will largely depend on 2 variables: the ability to artificially manufacture an appropriate substitute and the ability to streamline the tissue processing and demonstrate that it is safe.

ALLOGRAFT IN ACL LIGAMENT RECONSTRUCTION

ACL reconstruction surgery is currently the sixth most common orthopedic procedure nationwide with over 100,000 reconstructions per year.[38] More than 85% of the ACL reconstructions across the United States are done by surgeons who do less than 10 ACL reconstructions a year, so there is a lot of variation in graft choice and overall ACL surgical technique. BPTB autograft used to be the gold standard for graft choice, and according to the 2006 ACL study group conducted by JD Campbell, the hamstrings

(HS/BPTB) ratio was 2:3 but is likely equalizing to 1:1. Therefore, BPTB autograft is really no longer considered the gold standard. Over the last half decade, the range of graft choices available has exploded to encompass at least half a dozen different options ranging from bone-tendon-bone, hamstring, or quadriceps autograft to allograft bone-tendon-bone, Achilles tendon, tibialis anterior, tibialis posterior, or allograft hamstring.

Different patients have different needs and therefore should get different grafts. A collegiate division I football player has different needs and time constraints than a 40-year-old recreational athlete. Biologic healing has been studied in animals and these investigations largely show that while both allografts and autografts undergo similar stages of remodeling, allografts heal at a slower rate and at the same time points tend to be weaker. At 6 months, the autografts demonstrated better restraint to AP translation, twice the load-to-failure strength, a significant increase in graft size, and more small-diameter collagen fibrils (demonstrating remodeling). The allografts demonstrated a slower rate of incorporation and a prolonged inflammatory response.[39] ACL grafts undergo multiple stages of remodeling: graft necrosis, revascularization, fibroblast proliferation, and collagen synthesis. Multiple studies show that after these stages are complete, the implanted tissue is histologically similar to the native ACL.[39–42] Therefore, although the end result may be similar, there are clear implications for the rate of return to sport and rehabilitation based on graft choice.

Until recently, data comparing outcomes on primary ACL autograft and allograft have been similar.[43] However, more data are emerging with the MOON study sponsored in part by the National Institutes of Health. Some of the preliminary data from this trial were recently presented at the AOSSM 2008 in Orlando, FL, and showed that for young patients in the age group 10 to 19 years, the odds ratio of failure was 6.77 when compared with the autograft group.[4] In young athletes, BPTB autograft is preferred for a variety of reasons. Collegiate athletes have significant time constraints, and they can get back to sport as soon as 6 months. For young, small women athletes in whom the patella may not yield an adequate size graft, hamstring autograft is considered, unless they are competitive sprinters. Allograft reconstructions are reserved for older patients and for those who have a lower level of activity. Given the trend toward slower incorporation and potentially higher rates of failure in younger athletes, it is believed that allograft ACL will be less favorable in primary ACL reconstruction if the MOON data continue to show high failure rates among the young active population.

Authors' Preferences

The authors' approach to graft selection in ACL surgery is based on age and activity level. About 1/3 allograft usage in primary ACL reconstruction and 2/3 allograft usage in ACL revision cases are averaged. Both autograft and allograft are used routinely, but autograft is preferred in young competitive athletes. BPTB autograft is favored in most of the athletes but hamstring autograft is also done. The main concern with these athletes is the time to return to sport. With autograft surgery, a more aggressive approach is preferred with regard to postoperative rehabilitation, and in most cases, the athletes can be returned to full sports 2 to 3 months earlier than in allograft reconstruction. In older patients with ACL reconstruction, over the age of 40 years, allograft is preferred because the time constraint is not as vigorous, and these patients tend to do better with decreased morbidity without autograft harvest.

ALLOGRAFT IN MULTILIGAMENT RECONSTRUCTION

Knee dislocations are an uncommon, devastating injury. Usually at least 2 of the ligaments are disrupted, and there is concomitant injury to other structures of the knee such as the meniscus or articular cartilage. Nonsurgical treatment has been associated with poor outcomes, and therefore, a majority of these are treated surgically,[44] although relative indications for conservative treatment include older age, sedentary lifestyle, and debilitating medical or posttraumatic comorbidities. In these cases, conservative treatment with closed reduction and prolonged immobilization is preferred. It is worth mentioning that often these patients are still taken to the operating room to address loss of motion or persistent instability.[35]

The goal of reconstruction of the knee in knee dislocation is anatomic repair or reconstruction of all affected structures, that is, ligaments, menisci, and chondral injuries. Allograft is and will remain a good choice due to its availability, decreased surgical time (without harvest), and decreased donor-site morbidity, especially in a knee that is already traumatized.

Attempts at harvesting autograft, aside from being limited due to the surrounding trauma, are limited by available graft number as well as length. For example, to reconstruct a knee, potentially as many as 2 to 5 grafts are needed depending on the number of graft reconstructions and single- versus double-bundle considerations. This represents too many grafts to harvest from the patient, and therefore allograft remains a great option.

The goal with a knee dislocation, because of the amount of trauma involved, is not the same as that with a primary ACL reconstruction, and therefore the time constraints regarding return to sport are not an issue. In the case of multiligament reconstruction, autograft is really not an option, and allograft remains a good choice in the future evolution of multiligament reconstruction.

ALLOGRAFT IN MENISCUS TRANSPLANTATION

Meniscus function has been shown to be necessary for the preservation and normal function of the knee joint, contributing to nutrition, load transmission, and stability.[45] Current trends in knee surgery involve meniscal repair when possible, although there are a number of patients in whom meniscal tears are irreparable. Without a functional meniscus, these patients then are at risk for early arthritis in the affected knee.[46] First described in 1984 by Milachowski,[47] meniscal transplant is a reasonable option in these cases with young patients, good alignment, ligamentous stability, and minimal cartilage damage. The indications include relatively young patients who have previously undergone meniscectomy, complain of pain localized to the tibiofemoral compartment on the affected side, and have minimal chondrosis limited to the meniscal weight-bearing zone.[35]

Due to the lack of other options, allograft will continue to remain a good option for the patient described above. There is currently no autologous option for the meniscus. Additionally, there are no viable artificially manufactured menisci yet. Fresh-frozen and cryopreserved grafts encompass the majority of meniscal transplants today. Fresh meniscal allografts are not ideal secondary to the need for sizing and distribution, while freeze-dried allografts can shrink up to 66% in the process and therefore present a sizing problem in addition to the likelihood that the shrinkage is detrimental.[47,48]

The meniscal allografts have been shown in a sheep model to revascularize and heal within 6 weeks after implantation. At 48 weeks, the meniscus was completely revascularized and remodeled with cellular ingrowth and a newly formed collagenous structure.[47] Four weeks after implantation, DNA probe analysis showed that cells derived from the surrounding synovium repopulated the meniscus.[49] Clinically, second-look arthroscopy has confirmed that meniscal allografts heal after transplantation in the human knee.[50,51]

Authors' Preferences

The authors' clinical experience with meniscus transplantation has been favorable, and they believe that meniscus allografts at this point in time remain the only viable option for this procedure. Thirty-two patients were retrospectively reviewed after lateral meniscal transplantation at average 3.3-year follow-up. Ninety-six percent of the patients reported that overall function and activity level improved following surgery, short form 36-item (SF-36) scores were favorable, and follow-up radiographs showed no difference in joint-space narrowing compared with the contralateral side.[52] With regard to graft choice for meniscal transplantation, fresh-frozen allograft is preferred.

OSTEOCHONDRAL ALLOGRAFTS

There is no great option for the treatment of osteochondral defects. In large part, this is due to the fact that chondral defects do not heal themselves. Attempts to recreate cartilage with microfracture or abrasionplasty result in fibrocartilage not hyaline cartilage. Additionally, cartilage does not heal side to side, so with procedures like the osteoarticular transfer system or even allograft plugs, there may be some incorporation of the graft but not complete healing of the cartilage layer. Recent data from Gross and colleagues[53] with fresh osteochondral allograft show osteochondral allograft survival up to 25 years (average, 12 years) with retrieval studies. Factors associated with early failure include lack of chondrocyte viability and loss of matrix cationic staining. Late failures were associated with fracture through the graft, active and incomplete remodeling of the graft bone by the host bone, and resorption of the graft tissue by synovial inflammatory activity at the graft edges. Conversely, histologic factors associated with long-term graft survival included viable chondrocytes, functional preservation of matrix, and complete replacement of the graft bone with the host bone. Given the need for viable chondrocytes, the best options for osteochondral graft are either fresh allograft, as mentioned earlier, and cryopreserved grafts. Although the cells within the hyaline cartilage exist within an immunoprotective avascular environment and do not incite an immune response,[54,55] the bony portion does. This affects bone-to-bone healing and subsequent bony collapse. This risk is decreased with the processing that occurs with cryopreserved tissue, which may help with bony integration.

The bottom line is that fresh allograft is better for the chondral layer, because there are more chondrocytes, which are key to the graft survival, although this graft is worse in terms of the bony incorporation due to the immune response that can inhibit bony remodeling.

Fresh allograft needs to be harvested acutely and implanted within 7 days for best results, and therefore in most cases it is not user-friendly. Graft storage affects chondrocyte viability, and this has been studied. Cell viability and matrix characteristics with mean time to implantation 30 days after harvest and stored at 2° to 8° had a chondrocyte viability of 67%.[56] A sheep study looking for chondrocyte viability and the material properties of the matrix in femoral condyles after storage at 4° and up to 60 days involved measurement at time intervals. Mean chondrocyte viability decreased over time, at day 60 to 51%, with most of the nonviable chondrocytes at the superficial layer.[57] Cryopreserved allograft is processed with less immune antigens, so bony incorporation is better. The chondrocyte viability can be as high as 80%, but other studies have shown that relative to fresh allograft, cryopreserved grafts exhibit decreased chondrocyte viability and early articular degeneration.[58,59]

Clinical experience with fresh allograft has shown reasonable results. In one study, Bugbee and colleagues[60] reported on 97 patients with a mean follow-up of 50 months.

Sixty-one patients underwent grafting of 1 surface, 30 underwent 2-surface transplantation, and 5 patients had multiple chondral surfaces allografted. Success rates for mono- and bipolar transplants were 86%, whereas the success rate of multiple surfaces dropped to 53%. Poor outcome was associated with poor allograft fit, increase in affected surface area, and increase in surfaces involved. Clinical experience with cryopreserved allografts is less extensive, but clinical results are reasonable as well. Flynn and colleagues[61] reported on 17 knees with 70% success at a mean 4.2-year follow-up. Bakay and colleagues[62] reported on 33 cases with 69% excellent results at 19 months.

Authors' Preferences

Autograft transplantation is an option for chondral defects but is limited by size, given the need to harvest from another part of the knee as well as donor-site morbidity. Therefore, the main indication is a lesion size less 2 cm, and this is in agreement with that in the literature, which ranges from 2 to 3 cm as the cutoff size for allograft.[35,63] Fresh-frozen allograft is preferred. Given the lack of regenerative potential of hyaline cartilage in the knee, donor-site size constraints, and donor-site morbidity, allograft continues to be a good option for these types of lesions.

SUMMARY

Allografts have a definite place in sports medicine today. There are 2 large categories for allograft usage. The first category involves completely elective usage, such as in primary ACL reconstruction, where autograft can be harvested with very good results and the decision to use allograft is completely elective. In this case, the future role of allografts in sports will be largely dependent on the ability of the tissue procurement agencies and regulatory agencies to control the quality of the allograft, both in sterility and mechanical strength. The recent attention in the lay media about criminal activity and forging papers for potential tissue donors does not inspire confidence among the general population. Additionally, the fact that there are infectious agents such as prions, which we do not know much about and cannot test for, causes concern, not to mention the fact that we cannot test for all the other infectious disease agents we do not know about. Although the incidence of HIV and hepatitis transmission is very small, and most would say acceptable, bacterial infection is much more common, and deaths can occur from this type of infection, as mentioned in the case of the young man in Minnesota in 2001 who died of *Clostridium sordellii* after receiving an osteochondral allograft.

Recent evolution of ACL reconstruction surgical technique, with evidence that double-bundle ACL surgery is more anatomic and potentially better able to constrain the knee without as much concern of "overcapturing" it, has placed a premium on autograft harvesting, as this surgery requires 2 separate bundles. This can still be achieved with autograft but is a little bit trickier for those who do not perform many autograft harvest and double-bundle surgeries. In these cases, allograft may provide more flexibility in both graft size and length. The recent presentation at the AOSSM regarding the MOON trial is critical, as the preliminary data show allograft to be an independent risk factor for ACL failure with an odds ratio as high as 6.7. Again, until the full data and details emerge from this study, caution should be used in the interpretation of these data.

The authors' experience has been that in the high school and collegiate population with ACL reconstruction, returning to training and sport at certain time intervals is critical. Autograft allows this flexibility as remodeling occurs faster than with allograft, and for this reason, autograft is preferred in most of these situations. In cases where the physiologic load is much less, such as the MPFL, the ligament needs to withstand only 30N of force (compared with 2000N for the ACL) and largely serves as a checkrein. In these types of cases, allograft reconstruction may have an important role. The data, however, are pending. In this case, even with the transient weakening that the allograft undergoes during the ligamentization process, the graft construct is stronger than the everyday forces across that graft, so the rehabilitation timeline for allograft or autograft does not need to be different. Therefore, worry about "re-ligamentization" of the graft is not as much of an issue with regard to graft failure. Additionally, it has been the experience of the senior author (C.D.H.) that allograft incorporation is better in an "extra-articular" environment such as for the MPFL. Again, the data for this are pending.

The second category of allograft involves those cases where too much graft material is needed, and autograft harvest is therefore not a realistic option. This is the case for multiligament reconstruction, osteochondral allograft, and meniscal allograft transplantation as well. In this case, the decision to use allograft is not elective in the sense that there are no other options. For example, in a meniscal transplant, without the allograft, transplant is not possible. In this case, the risk-benefit equation is the benefit of meniscal transplant versus the risk of infection; this differs from the case of the primary ACL, where either way the ACL surgery can be done.

Although the screening process for infectious disease continues to improve and the incidence of infection is very low, the future cannot be predicted. Two decades ago the AIDS epidemic or the pervasiveness of hepatitis could not have been predicted. Although the screening processes have evolved to manage these diseases, this is always in reaction to cases that have already occurred. Today, there are concerns about prion disease and other diseases such as Chagas disease, West Nile virus, and other somewhat obscure, but potentially significant, outbreaks. With the implementation of newer screening tools such as PCR and NAT, and in the absence of another deadly pandemic, allografts will continue to have a prominent place in sports medicine.

New technology is constantly on the horizon. Genetic engineering and stem cell research may provide a way in the future to regrow ligaments and menisci. In these cases, assuming that the price for technology is not prohibitive, these pseudo-autografts will be a good alternative to the allograft. There is no indication that this will be commercially available in the near future, but it is worth comment, nonetheless. With regard to cartilage technology, attempts to regrow cartilage will, in large part, depend on the ability to manufacture scaffolds with appropriate growth factors and matrix population.

REFERENCES

1. U.S. Census Bureau. Statistical abstract of the United States 2001, No. 168, organ transplants and grafts, 1990–2000. Available at: http://www.census.gov/prod/2002pubs/01statab/health.pdf. Accessed March 2002.
2. Gocke D. Tissue donor selection and safety. Clin Orthop Relat Res 2005;435:22.
3. Leever RS. 2006 AOSSM orthopaedic surgical procedure survey on allografts. AOSSM 2006.
4. Kaeding CC, PA, Aros BC, et al. Independent predictors of ACL reconstruction failure from the MOON prospective longitudinal cohort. AOSSM 2008 Final Program, 2008:121.
5. Suarez LS, RJ. Overview of procurement, processing, and sterilization of soft tissue allografts for sports medicine. Sports Med Arthrosc Rev 2007;15:106.

6. Tomford WW, MH. Bone banking: update on methods and materials. Orthop Clin North Am 1999;30:565.
7. Harner CD, OE, Irrgang JJ, et al. Allograft versus autograft anterior cruciate ligament reconstruction: 3–5 year outcome. Clin Orthop 1996;324:134.
8. Lephart SM, KM, Harner CD, et al. Quadriceps strength and functional capacity after anterior cruciate ligament reconstruction: patellar tendon autograft versus allograft. Am J Sports Med 1993;21:738.
9. Boyce T, EJ, Scarborough N. Allograft bone: the influence of processing on safety and performance. Orthop Clin North Am 1999;30.
10. Vangsness CJ. Soft-tissue allograft processing controversies. J Knee Surg 2006; 19:215.
11. (CDC) CfDCaP. About tissue transplants. Available at: www.cdc.gov/ncidod/ dhqp/tissuetransplantsFAQ.html. 2006.
12. Vangsness CT, GI, Mills R, et al. Allograft transplantation in the knee: tissue regulation, procurement, processing, and sterilization. Am J Sports Med 2003; 31:474.
13. General OoI: oversight of tissue banking. Available at: www.fda.gov/ohrms/ dockets/ac/01/briefing/3736b2_01.pdf. 2001.
14. Administration UFaD. Guidance for industry: eligibility determination for donors of human cells tissues and cellular and tissue based products: final rule. Available at: www.fda.gov/cber/gdlns/tissdonor.htm. 2007.
15. Maclean V. American Association of Tissue Banks: standards for tissue banking. American Association of Tissue Banks, October 2006.
16. LeDell KH, LR, Danila RN, et al. Public health dispatch update: unexplained deaths following knee surgery—Minnesota 2001. MMWR - Morb Mortal Wkly Rep 2001;50:1080.
17. Prevention CfDCa: Notice to readers: unexplained deaths following knee surgery—Minnesota. MMWR Morb Mortal Wkly Rep 2001;50:1035.
18. Archibald LK, JD, Kainer MA. Update: allograft-associated bacterial infections— United States. MMWR Morb Mortal Wkly Rep 2002;51:207.
19. Administration UFaD. Recall of human tissue, biomedical tissue services LTD. Rockville (MD): Food and Drug Administration; 2006.
20. Administration UFaD. Recall of human tissue intended for transplantations. Fort Lee (NJ): Food and Drug Administration; 2006.
21. Administration UFaD. FDA public health notification: donor referral services. Rockville (MD): Food and Drug Administration; 2006.
22. Marchione M. Patient got tainted cadaver tissue. ABC News, 2006.
23. Vangsness CT, TM, Joyce MJ, et al. Soft tissue for allograft reconstruction of the human knee: a survey of the American Association of Tissue Banks. Am J Sports Med 1996;24:230.
24. Organizations AoOP. AOPO accredited OPO's. Association of Organ Procurement Organizations, 2006.
25. Branam BR, JD. Allografts in knee surgery. Orthopedics 2007;30:925.
26. Dodd RY, Stramer SL. Current prevalence and incidence of infectious disease markers and estimated window-period risk in the American Red Cross blood donor population. Transfusion 2002;42:975.
27. Buck BE, MT. Human bone and tissue allografts. Preparation and safety. Clin Orthop 1994;303:8.
28. Zou S, DR, Stramer SL, Tissue Safety Study Group. Probability of viremia with HBV, HCV, HIV, and HTLV among tissue donors in the United States. N Engl J Med 2004;351:751.

29. Buck BE, MT, Brown MD. Bone transplantation and human immunodeficiency virus: an estimate of risk of acquired immunodeficiency syndrome (AIDS). Clin Orthop 1989;240:129.

30. Simonds RJ, HS, Hurwitz RL, et al. Transmission of human immunodeficiency virus type 1 from seronegative organ and tissue donor. N Engl J Med 1992;326: 726.

31. (CDC) CfDC. Transmission of HIV through bone transplantation: case report and public health recommendations. MMWR Morb Mortal Wkly Rep 1988;37: 597.

32. Tomford W. Transmission of disease through transplantation of musculoskeletal allografts. Journal of Bone and Joint Surgery–American edition 1995;77A:1742.

33. Shelton W. Arthroscopic allograft surgery of the knee and shoulder: indications, techniques, and risks. Arthroscopy 2003;19:67.

34. Tugwell BD, WI, Thomas AR, et al. Hepatitis C (HCV) transmission of tissue and organ recipients from an antibody-negative donor. In: The Interscience Conference on Antimicrobial Agents and Chemotherapy. San Diego, 2002.

35. Rihn JA, HC. The use of musculoskeletal allograft tissue in knee surgery. Arthroscopy 2003;19:51.

36. Shelton WR, TS, Dukes AD, et al. Use of allografts in knee reconstruction: I. Basic science aspects and current status. J Am Acad Orthop Surg 1998;6:165.

37. Fideler BM, VC, Moore T, et al. Effects of gamma irradiation on the human immunodeficiency virus. A study in frozen human bone-patellar ligament-bone grafts obtained from infected cadavers. Journal of Bone and Joint Surgery–American edition 1994;76A:1032.

38. Surgery. ABoO: Research Committee Report: Diplomatic Newsletter. American Board of Orthopaedic Surgery, 2004.

39. Jackson DW, GE, Arnoczky SP, et al. Freeze dried anterior cruciate ligament allografts: preliminary studies in a goat model. Am J Sports Med 1987;15:295.

40. Arnoczky SP, WR, Ashlock MA. Replacement of the anterior cruciate ligament using a patellar tendon allograft: an experimental study. Journal of Bone and Joint Surgery–American edition 1986;68:376.

41. Drez DJ, DJ, Holden JP, et al. Anterior cruciate ligament reconstruction using bone patellar tendon bone allografts: a biological and biomechanical evaluation in goats. Am J Sports Med 1991;19:256.

42. Shino K, KT, Hirose H, et al. Replacement of the anterior cruciate ligament by an allogenic tendon graft: an experimental study in the dog. JBJS Br 1984;66:672.

43. Jackson DW, CJ, Simon TM. Biologic incorporation of allograft anterior cruciate ligament replacements. Clin Orthop 1996;324:126.

44. Richter M, BU, Wippermann B, et al. Comparison of surgical repair or reconstruction of the cruciate ligaments versus nonsurgical treatment in patients with traumatic knee dislocations. Am J Sports Med 2002;30:718.

45. Aagaard H, VR. Function of the normal meniscus and consequences of meniscus resection. Scand J Med Sci Sports 1999;9:134.

46. Fairbank T. Knee changes after meniscectomy. Journal of Bone and Joint Surgery–British edition 1948;30:664.

47. Milachowski KA, WK, Wirth CJ. Homologous meniscus transplantation: experimental and clinical results. Int Orthop 1989;13:1.

48. Wirth CJ, PG, Milachowski KA, et al. Long term results of meniscal allograft transplantation. Am J Sports Med 2002;30:174.

49. Jackson DW, WJ, Simon TM. Cell survival after transplantation of fresh meniscal allografts: DNA probe analysis in a goat model. Am J Sports Med 1993;21:540.

50. Van Arkel ER, DBH. Human meniscal transplantation. Preliminary results at 2–5 year follow-up. Journal of Bone and Joint Surgery–British edition 1995;77:589.
51. Verdonk R. Alternative treatments for meniscal injuries. Journal of Bone and Joint Surgery–British edition 1997;79:866.
52. Sekiya JK, WR, Groff YJ, et al. Clinical outcomes following isolated lateral meniscal allograft transplantation. Arthroscopy 2006;22:771.
53. Gross AE, OO, Kim W, et al. Fresh osteochondral allografts for posttraumatic knee defects: long term follow-up. Clin Orthop Relat Res 2008;466:1863.
54. Langer F, GA. Immunogenicity of allograft articular cartilage. JBJS Am 1974;56:297.
55. Oakeshott RD, FI, Pritzker KP, et al. A clinical and histologic analysis of failed fresh osteochondral allografts. Clin Orthop 1988;233:283.
56. Pearsall AW, TA, Hester RB, et al. Chondrocyte viability in refrigerated osteochondral allografts used for transplantation within the knee. Chondrocyte viability in refrigerated osteochondral allografts used for transplantation within the knee. Am J Sports Med 2004;32:125.
57. Williams RJ, DJ, Chen CT. Chondrocyte survival and material properties of hypothermically stored cartilage: an evaluation of tissue used for osteochondral allograft transplantation. Am J Sports Med 2004;32:132.
58. Malinin TI, MW, Lo HK, et al. Cryopreservation of articular cartilage. Ultrastructural observations and long-term results of experimental distal femoral transplantation. Clin Orthop Relat Res 1994;303:18.
59. Ohlendorf C, TW, Mankin HJ. Chondrocyte survival in cryopreserved osteochondral articular cartilage. J Orthop Res 1996;14:413.
60. Bugbee WD, CF. Osteochondral allograft transplantation. Clin Sports Med 1999;18:67.
61. Flynn JM, SD, Mankin HJ. Osteoarticular allografts to treat distal femoral osteonecrosis. Clin Orthop 1994;303:38.
62. Bakay A, CL, Papp G, et al. Osteochondral resurfacing of the knee joint with allograft: clinical analysis of 33 cases. Int Orthop 1998;22:277.
63. Gross A. Repair of cartilage defects in the knee. J Knee Surg 2002;15:167.

Index

Note: Page numbers of article titles are in **boldface** type.

A

Achilles tendon allografts, 191, 192
  for anterior cruciate ligament reconstruction. See *Anterior cruciate ligament reconstruction.*
Allograft tissue, processed, storage of, 197–198
Allograft(s), Achilles tendon, 191, 192
  augmentation versus reconstruction of medial collateral ligament using, **303–310**
  autograft versus, for ligament reconstruction, 215–216
  biologic incorporation of, 217
  bone-patellar tendon-bone, 191, 192, 315
  clinical outcomes of, 217–218
  concerns about safety of, 329–330, 331–332
  concerns and considerations in use of, 215
  donor of, screening of, 224
  donor-site morbidity and, 216
  for anterior cruciate ligament reconstruction, 216, 218
    for young athlete, 217–218, 219
  for primary anterior cruciate ligament reconstruction, **223–244**
    advantages/disadvantages of, 226–227
    biologic incorporation of, 227–228
    risk of disease transmission and, 225–226
  fresh-frozen, for massive defects, 219
  future of, in sports medicine, **329–342**
  gamma irradiation of, 195, 224–225
  in anterior cruciate ligament reconstruction, 334–335
  in meniscus transplantation, 336–337
  in multiligament reconstruction, 335–336
  in orthopedic surgery, advantages of, 203
  incorporation of, biology of, **203–214**
  increasing use in orthopedic surgery, 223
  infection as concern in use of, 331, 332–333
  long-term durability of, factors influencing, 219
  most common, 216
  musculoskeletal. See *Musculoskeletal allografts.*
  osteochondral. See *Osteochondral allografts.*
  procurement, sterilization, and storage of, 191, 193
  procurement and use of, history of, 330
  soft tissue. See *Soft tissue allografts.*
  sterilization of, 224–225
  tibialis, 191, 193
  used in knee reconstruction, 191, 192
  what do we really know about? **215–222**

Clin Sports Med 28 (2009) 341–347
doi:10.1016/S0278-5919(09)00017-9
0278-5919/09/$ – see front matter
sportsmed.theclinics.com

Moving?

Make sure your subscription moves with you!

To notify us of your new address, find your **Clinics Account Number** (located on your mailing label above your name), and contact customer service at:

E-mail: elspcs@elsevier.com

800-654-2452 (subscribers in the U.S. & Canada)
314-453-7041 (subscribers outside of the U.S. & Canada)

Fax number: 314-523-5170

Elsevier Periodicals Customer Service
11830 Westline Industrial Drive
St. Louis, MO 63146

*To ensure uninterrupted delivery of your subscription, please notify us at least 4 weeks in advance of move.

ELSEVIER